William M. Beneke / Robert A. Hancock

Study Guide / Workbook

ABNORMAL PSYCHOLOGY

Spencer A. Rathus / Jeffrey S. Nevid

Prentice Hall   Englewood Cliffs, New Jersey   07632

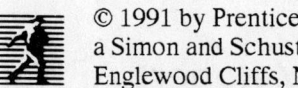 © 1991 by Prentice-Hall, Inc.
a Simon and Schuster Company
Englewood Cliffs, New Jersey 07632

Production supervision: Karen Winget
Buyers: Debra Kesar/Mary Ann Gloriande
Supplemental acquisitions editor: Sharon Chambliss
Acquisitions editor: Susan Finnemore
Cover designer: Meryl Poweski

Printed in the United States of America

10 9 8 7 6 5 4 3 2 1

ISBN 0-13-005364-3

Prentice-Hall International (UK) Limited, *London*
Prentice-Hall of Australia Pty. Limited, *Sydney*
Prentice-Hall of Canada Inc., *Toronto*
Prentice-Hall Hispanoamericana, S.A., *Mexico*
Prentice-Hall of India Private Limited, *New Delhi*
Prentice-Hall of Japan, Inc., *Tokyo*
Simon & Schuster Asia Pte. Ltd., *Singapore*
Editora Prentice-Hall do Brasil, Ltda., *Rio de Janeiro*

Contents

Preface

A Message to Students

First of all, thank you for reading this. Authors, that's us, write study guides in the hope that those study guides will help you, the student, learn more, faster. We write them with a specific strategy, based upon sound psychological principles, for using the study guide in mind. We believe, and in some cases can prove, that using your study guide according to that strategy will produce more effective and efficient study. Our, and your instructor's, bottom line is that you learn more, more efficiently. Your bottom line is better grades with less effort. Nevertheless, our efforts to develop an effective strategy and write a better study guide will be wasted unless you use this study guide properly. That is, you need to read the instructions, the stuff that follows. So thanks for reading this "how to" section and making our efforts worthwhile.

An Outline of This Study Guide

This study guide is broken into chapters, one chapter of the study guide for each chapter in your text. Within each chapter of this study guide, there are seven sections. The first section is the **OVERVIEW**. To no one's surprise, in this section, we will provide you with an overview or survey of what is in each chapter in your text.

The next section is the **CHAPTER OUTLINE WITH LESSONS & LEARNING OBJECTIVES**. This section, as its name implies, does three things. The **Chapter Outline** provides an outline of the chapter in your text. The numbered **Learning Objectives** tell you what information is important to know. Knowing these objectives will not only tell you what is important but also make you a more active reader by directing your attention to the most critical information in your text. The Learning Objectives are then grouped together into **Lessons**. A Lesson represents a chunk of text material you should read and study, at one time. [In fact, one of us (RAH) wanted to call the Lessons "Chapter Chunks" but the other of us (WMB) objected.] We have gone through your text and grouped together those learning objectives which have a common theme. The title for each lesson is a brief description of that theme.

The third section is the "meat" of the study guide. For each Lesson, there is a **Mastering Lesson** section containing a summary and a term matching exercise. The summary in the Mastering Lesson section will give you an overview of the text for that lesson and, perhaps more importantly, our "helpful hints" on how and what to study and learn. That is, in the mastering lesson summaries, we will tell you how we would go about studying and learning the material in your text.

The fourth section, **PRACTICE EXAM**, contains a true-false exam and a multiple-choice exam. For each learning objective in the chapter, there is one true-false question and one multiple-choice question.

Key terms from your chapter and the page on which you can find them are listed in **TERMS AND CONCEPTS**. In the section **TYING THINGS TOGETHER**, you will find two or three activities or questions. Completing the exercises and answering the questions will tie together major sections of the textbook chapter. Some people call these type of activities and questions "Study Questions." Our purpose in including them is to give you a way to integrate the specific information contained in the lessons back to the issues discussed in the Overview. Writing out answers or completing the exercise and then going over them with your instructor is the best possible way to make sense of the vast amount of information contained in the textbook. Doing this will enable you to get the most out of the class you are taking. The final section of the study guide, **ANSWERS**, contains answers for the Practice Exam.

How to Use This Study Guide

Whenever you attempt to learn or do anything, the first thing to do is to get a "rough idea" or general overview of what you will be learning or doing. Therefore, the very first thing you need to do, before you start reading your text, is to read the **OVERVIEW** of your study guide. The OVERVIEW will provide you with a basic framework for understanding and learning what is in your text. You will find that reading your text will be easier if you have some idea of what to expect.

Once, you have read the OVERVIEW and know what to expect, you should read the **CHAPTER OUTLINE WITH LESSONS & LEARNING OBJECTIVES**. The learning objectives here will provide the answer to the question "what stuff do I need to know?" Remember, knowing these objectives will tell you what is important and make you a more active and effective reader.

Finally, jump ahead in your study guide to the section entitled **Mastering Lesson 1**. Under Mastering Lesson 1, there is a brief lesson summary. Read this lesson summary. In this lesson summary, we provide an overview of the lesson and tell you how we would go about learning that lesson.

Once you have read the lesson summary for the first lesson, you should then <u>read</u> those pages in <u>your textbook</u> indicated by Lesson 1, taking reading notes in a separate notebook as you read. [We know that most of you won't take reading notes but we also know that taking them is a good idea.]

Once you have read the pages for Lesson 1, return to the study guide and **Mastering Lesson 1**. Under Mastering Lesson 1, you will find a list of the key terms and concepts for mastering the Learning Objectives for this lesson. Your job is to match each key term and concept with the appropriate definition or description. This will give you an immediate opportunity to determine what you have learned.

A word to the wise: it is very tempting not to do the actual matching but simply read the terms and concepts and the definitions and descriptions. You may find a little voice in your head saying "I know what the answer to that is" or "I remember reading that" and you go on without actually finding and indicating your answer. If you do that, you will find yourself thinking the same things on exam days but you won't be able to pull out the answer. To remember things, you have to practice remembering them.

Once, you've completed matching the key terms/concepts with their definitions/descriptions, the best thing to do is to check to see if your answers are correct by checking back to your textbook or the notes you took while reading your text. Many students refuse to do this, so we have provided an answer key for each lesson at the end of each chapter. Where you have made errors, you should immediately refer back to your text. In the section **TERMS AND CONCEPTS**, we have listed each of the key terms and concepts in the chapter listed alphabetically with a textbook page reference. Once you have corrected your work take a brief study break from Abnormal Psychology.

After your study break is over, you need to repeat this procedure for the next Lesson. Go to Mastering Lesson 2, read the summary, find the textbook page reference for this lesson, and then read those pages in your textbook. After you have read the pages for Lesson 2, jump back to the matching for Mastering Lesson 2 and complete that section. Repeat the procedure until you have completed all of the Lessons for a chapter. At this time, take a break from studying abnormal psychology of at least one hour.

When you return from your break, you will be ready to face a test of what you really know. First, read the Summary, located at the end of the chapter, in your text. This will refresh your memory and make it easier to remember information on the exams to follow. Next, complete the section in your study guide called **PRACTICE EXAM**. This section consists of two exams, a true-false exam and a multiple-choice exam. On each exam, there will be one question focused on each Learning Objective.

You should take these Practice Exams in the same way you take classroom tests. Completing a practice exam is the same as having a dress rehearsal before a performance or a conducting scrimmage before a game. The Practice Exams are an opportunity to check your knowledge under test-like conditions. Take them in a quiet place with your textbook closed. Once you've completed the Practice Exams, check your answers against the answer key we have provided.

How to Read a Textbook

Reading a textbook to extract information requires a rather peculiar kind of reading. The best way, that is, the way that takes the least amount of time to produce the most learning is read and take notes. At first, this method will seem very time consuming but if done properly it can save you the agony of rereading and rereading and rereading.

The place to start is with a standard notebook, one for each textbook. [Yes, you're going to learn why notebooks were invented.] At the top of each page, one to a page, write out the Learning Objectives for each chapter in order. Then, as you read the chapter, stop at the end of each section where you find information important to a Learning Objective. In the top half of every page, briefly summarize that information by writing a note to yourself, not to anyone else. Once, you have enough information for a Learning Objective, write a brief summary of that information to yourself.

What you have produced by doing this is a set of reading notes. So that anytime you need some information, you can go directly to these notes which will help remind you what you have read. Going over these reading notes in preparation for a Final Exam will be easier, faster, and ensure greater success than pulling the "all nighter" to reread the text.

Finally, if you have any comments on or suggestions for study guides, please write us and share your ideas.

Robert A. Hancock
Assistant Professor of Psychology

William M. Beneke
Professor of Psychology

Department of Social and Behavioral Sciences
Lincoln University of Missouri
Jefferson City, MO 65102

Acknowledgments

Thanks to Wayne Spohr and Don Hull of Prentice Hall for their recommendations to get us involved in this project. Thanks to Sharon Chambliss, our editor, for working so hard on our behalf. Finally, thanks to William Chally, for his technical advice on the computer hardware and software that enabled us to make this thing look so good.

1 What is Abnormal Psychology?

OVERVIEW

This chapter introduces the field of abnormal psychology; it is divided into three major sections. The first defines and illustrates the concept of abnormal behavior.

The second major section traces the history of abnormal behavior. You will quickly come to appreciate that the way society viewed abnormal behavior was a major determinant of how society treated mental illness. This is still true today. Contemporary psychologists have developed several different models of abnormal behavior, and the second section ends with an introduction to seven major viewpoints.

The final section explores research methods used in abnormal psychology. Much of our knowledge of abnormal behavior is the result of application of scientific method. This section provides a brief review of scientific method and then elaborates on specific research methods that are widely used to study abnormal behavior and its treatment.

CHAPTER OUTLINE, LESSONS & LEARNING OBJECTIVES

Lesson 1. Defining abnormal behavior. (1-5)
DEFINING ABNORMAL BEHAVIOR. (1-5)
1. List and briefly describe the six criteria that define abnormal behavior. Be able to apply these criteria to examples of behavior by labelling them as normal or abnormal.

Lesson 2. The history of abnormal behavior. (5-12)
ABNORMAL BEHAVIOR IN HISTORICAL PERSPECTIVE. (5-18)
2. Describe the demonological view of abnormal behavior as it appeared in ancient and medieval times.
3. Summarize the contributions of Hippocrates, Galen, Weyer, Pasteur, Griesinger and Kraepelin to the development of medical science and its view of abnormal behavior.
4. Describe the development of treatment centers for abnormal behavior from asylums through the mental hospital.
5. Summarize the impact of the reform movement and the use of moral therapy on the treatment of abnormal behavior. Focus on the contributions of Pussin, Pinel, Rush and Dix.
6. Discuss the factors associated with the current exodus from mental hospitals in the United States.

Lesson 3. Contemporary models. (12-18)
7. Describe the viewpoints of seven contemporary models of abnormal behavior.

Lesson 4. Applying scientific methods to the study of abnormal behavior. (18-22)
RESEARCH METHODS IN ABNORMAL PSYCHOLOGY. (18-30)
8. State the objectives of a scientific approach to abnormal behavior.
9. Describe the steps involved in the scientific method.
10. Describe the method of naturalistic observation and discuss its values and limitations.
11. Understand the importance of drawing representative samples from target populations.
12. Define correlational research and discuss its value and limitations.
13. Describe longitudinal research methods.

Lesson 5. Experimental and epidemiological methods in the study of abnormal behavior. (22-27)
14. Summarize the purpose and essential features of the experimental method.
15. Tell how experimenters control for expectations of researchers and research subjects.
16. Name and identify three types of experimental validity.
17. Describe the values and limitations of quasi-experiments.
18. Describe the nature of epidemiological method, including its value and limitations.

Lesson 6. Studying abnormal behavior in individuals. (27-30)
19. Discuss the value and limitations of the case-study method.
20. Describe single-subject experimental designs and explain how they overcome some limitations of the case-study method.

Mastering Lesson 1. Defining abnormal behavior. (1-5)

You should immediately notice that abnormal behavior is defined more narrowly in psychology than it is in common English. Six criteria are used to decide if a behavior is abnormal. Mastery of this objective requires that you learn the six criteria and how to tell if a behavior meets each of them. Resist the temptation to rely on your everyday intuitions! You must analyze a behavior in terms of all six criteria and then make a logical decision. Do the matching exercise below to be sure that you are familiar with the criteria. Then review the examples in the text to be sure that you understand why the authors called each example normal or abnormal.

Match the following terms and concepts with the correct definition or description or explanation.

1. __ abnormal psychology
2. __ dangerous behavior
3. __ faulty perception of reality
4. __ maladaptive behavior
5. __ severe personal distress
6. __ socially unacceptable
7. __ unusual behavior

a. hallucinations and delusions
b. studies the description, causes, and treatment of abnormal behavior
c. anxiety, fear, and depression
d. uncommon or statistically deviant behavior
e. normal behavior in one culture can be abnormal in another
f. directed at oneself or others
g. limits our ability to function

Mastering Lesson 2. The history of abnormal behavior. (5-12)

In learning the material for the objectives in this lesson, you will quickly discover that the history of treatment of abnormal behavior seems a bit like a horror movie. Pay attention to the relationship between how abnormal behavior was viewed and the kinds of treatment that were used. In studying the reading information in this lesson learn to associate a particular approach (demonological, for instance) with its characteristic view of causes and treatment methods. Learn what major contributions were made by some major individuals and try to understand how these contributions changed society's view of abnormal behavior and how it was treated. You should practice associating ideas in both directions: person--> contributions and contributions-->persons. Your professor may choose to ask you to do either or both at examination time. The matching section below will help you form many needed associations.

Match the following terms and concepts with the correct definition or description or explanation.

1. __ asylums
2. __ Benjamin Rush
3. __ deinstitutionalization
4. __ demonological model
5. __ Dorthea Dix
6. __ Emil Kraeplin
7. __ exorcism
8. __ Galen
9. __ Hippocrates
10. __ humors in the body
11. __ Jean-Baptiste Pussin
12. __ John Weyer
13. __ Louis Pasteur
14. __ medical model
15. __ medieval view
16. __ moral therapy
17. __ Phillipe Pinel
18. __ Wilhelm Griesinger

a. abnormal behavior is a symptom of possession by evil spirits

b. believed humoral imbalance accounted for abnormal behavior

c. continued humane treatment at La Bicetre, early proponent of "talking therapies"

d. explanation of abnormal behavior that relies on the supernatural or divine

e. abnormal behavior explained by underlying biological or biochemical disorder

f. restore normal behavior by providing humane treatment in a relaxed, positive environment

g. believed madness was caused by engorgement of blood vessels

h. medieval treatment of choice for abnormal behavior

i. abnormal behavior results from disease of brain

j. early institutions for housing mentally ill

k. crusader whose efforts led to establishment of 32 mental hospitals in the USA

l. dementia praecox and manic depressive psychosis were two groups of mental disorder

m. first in the modern era to treat incurably insane with kindness

n. expanded upon teaching of Hippocrates; discovered arteries carried blood

o. made discoveries that supported the medical model view of physical disorders

p. Renaissance physician, argued that abnormal behavior was due to physical causes

q. phlegm, black bile, yellow bile and blood

r. trend resulting from the community mental health centers act and tranquilizers

3

Mastering Lesson 3. Contemporary models. (12-18)

Contemporary views of abnormal are ather diverse. Contemporary disagreements about the causes and treatment of abonormal behavior occur for two reasons. Different contemporary views are tied to different historical views and arose out of different disciplines. These views are trying to explain the same abnormal behaviors in different ways. Their <u>names</u> are major hints that tell you what each focuses on as it tries to identify the causes of abnormal behavior. As you learn about the contemporary models, try to relate information in this lesson to the previous one. All of the contemporary models are set in the historical context you just learned about. This is a key lesson. It is expanded in Chapter 2, and forms the framework for much of the remainder of the text.

Match the following terms and concepts with the correct definition or description or explanation.

1. __ behavior therapy
2. __ cognitive perspective
3. __ eclectic models
4. __ Ellis and Beck
5. __ humanistic-existential perspective
6. __ learning perspective
7. __ medical model
8. __ psychoanalysis
9. __ psychodynamic model
10. __ Rogers and Maslow
11. __ Sigmund Freud
12. __ social learning theory
13. __ sociocultural perspective
14. __ Watson, Skinner and Pavlov

a. major behaviorists
b. psychologists of humanistic persuasion
c. cognitive psychologists
d. abnormal behavior is caused by stress resulting from poverty and lack of opportunity
e. abnormal behavior is learned in relatively unique (and undesirable) situations
f. abnormal behavior due to inappropriate and unrealistic thoughts, expectations and attitudes
g. combines views of multiple models to explain abnormal behavior
h. abnormal behavior is symptomatic of an inner cause or "disease state"
i. a learning perspective emphasizing personal values, expectancies and views of others
j. psychodynamic model developed by Sigmund Freud
k. abnormal behavior results from subjective experience of roadblocks to self-actualization
l. a central figure in the psychodynamic perspective
m. application of learning principles to overcome psychological problems
n. abnormal behavior results from unconscious psychological conflicts

Mastering Lesson 4. Applying scientific methods to the study of abnormal behavior. (18-22)

This lesson serves primarily to review what you probably have learned elsewhere about the goals of science and scientific methods. A good working knowledge of this lesson will serve you well in future chapters. Also in this lesson are two research methods, naturalistic observation and longitudinal studies. Both methods are examples of correlational research. They can yield considerable valuable information, but they cannot determine causal relationships. Often, results of correlational studies appear to suggest a cause--effect relationship. Be wary of jumping to that kind of conclusion. Correlational studies fail to rule out possible effects of other causal factors. The matching section that follows will help you relearn a bit about scientific methods.

Match the following terms and concepts with the correct definition or description or explanation.

1. __	causal relationships	a.	inverse relationship
2. __	control	b.	two events in sequence where the first determines the second
3. __	correlation		
4. __	description	c.	description, explanation, prediction and control
5. __	explanation	d.	theories help us do this
6. __	longitudinal study	e.	altering causal factors to prevent development of abnormal behavior would be an example
7. __	naturalistic observation		
8. __	negative correlation	f.	two variables change in same direction
9. __	objectives of science	g.	unobtrusively observing behavior as it happens in the natural environment
10. __	population		
11. __	positive correlation	h.	formulate question, develop and test hypothesis, draw conclusions
12. __	prediction		
13. __	research sample	i.	study of the same individuals over a long period of time
14. __	scientific method		
15. __	significant differences	j.	the subjects in a research project
		k.	the group to whom a researcher wishes to generalize research findings
		l.	discovery of facts that anticipate the occurrence of events
		m.	differences that are statistically unlikely to be due to chance
		n.	in science, should be clear, unbiased and based on careful observation
		o.	measure of relationship between two variables

Mastering Lesson 5. Experimental and epidemiological methods in the study of abnormal behavior. (22-27)

Experimental methods are among the most powerful tools of science because of their ability to establish causal (cause-effect) relationships. This lesson begins with a review of the essential features of experimental methods. In abnormal psychology, expectations of both subjects and experimenters represent special problems, particularly for studies investigating therapies. Single-blind and double-blind placebo-control studies are specific kinds of experiments that control for expectancy effects.

In this lesson, you also will learn that you cannot always take results of experiments as gold-standard facts. Experiments differ in quality. This quality is represented as validity, or more precisely as three kinds of validity. The extent to which you should trust (believe in) experimental results depends upon that experiment's internal, external and construct validities. Pay attention to what these are and also to the differences in how problems with each type of validity should affect your view of the results of an experiment.

The use of experimental methods in applied settings is often difficult. Sometimes external constraints posed by the situation make true experiments impossible. Researchers often rely on research methods that use many (but not all) of the features of experimental methods in quasi-experiments. Pay attention to how quasi-experiments differ from experiments and how these differences should affect ones trust.

Epidemiological research method appears in this lesson because of its location in the chapter. It is not an experimental research method at all. It is an important means of estimating the incidence of various behavior disorders. The following matching section will help you review all of this. Completing the matching also will help you become more fluent in using the important terms and concepts related to the application of scientific method.

Match the following terms and concepts with the correct definition or description or explanation.

1. __ analogue study
2. __ construct validity
3. __ dependent variable
4. __ double-blind
5. __ epidemiological method
6. __ experimental method
7. __ experimental validity
8. __ external validity
9. __ independent variable
10. __ internal validity
11. __ placebo
12. __ quasi-experiment
13. __ random assignment
14. __ random sampling
15. __ selection factor
16. __ single-blind
17. __ stratified random sampling

a. increases external validity
b. construct, internal and external
c. common in epidemiological studies
d. manipulated by the scientist; the "cause" in cause-effect relationships
e. measured by the scientist; the "effect" in cause-effect relationships
f. eliminates the selection factor as an explanation for experimental results
g. differences in subjects between experimental and control groups
h. design that controls for subject and experimenter expectancy effects
i. concerned with incidence of abnormal behavior in different population groups but not with specific cause-effect relationships
j. extent to which experimental results can be generalized
k. an inactive manipulation used to control for subject expectations
l. requires control for possible confounding factors
m. a research method that often has questionable external validity
n. treatment effect results from theoretical mechanism represented in independent variable
o. an experimental method that lacks random assignment
p. subjects are kept uninformed about the treatments they receive
q. directly manipulates an independent variable to discover causal relationships

Mastering Lesson 6. Studying abnormal behavior in individuals. (27-30)

Much of what we know about abnormal behavior has come from the study of individuals. After all, one criterion for labelling behavior as abnormal is that the behavior is unusual. Then too, the learning model of abnormal behavior suggests that relatively unique learning histories may come into play. One way to attempt to get at all of this is the case study. Pay attention to what the case study is and what kinds of information it yields. You will notice (quickly, I trust) that case studies are rich in information about all sorts of things in a subject's life history but very short on scientific rigor (you should try to identify shortcomings in terms of the concepts you have already learned in this chapter). The main value of the case study is therefore to stimulate research questions that could be followed up using more powerful research methods.

Single-case experimental designs represent one way of overcoming the limitations of case studies. In learning about the two kinds of single-case experimental designs, you should focus on what these designs are and on how they attempt to establish <u>internal validity</u> of the experiment.

Match the following terms and concepts with the correct definition or description or explanation.

1. ___ case study
2. ___ generalization limits its value
3. ___ multiple-baseline design
4. ___ requires returning to baseline conditions
5. ___ reversal design
6. ___ single-case experimental design

a. multiple-baseline design
b. reversal design
c. A-B-A-B
d. multiple-baseline and reversal are major types
e. rich in clinical material but lacking in scientific rigor
f. establishes baselines for two or more behaviors and applies treatment at different times

PRACTICE EXAMS

Exam 1. (true-false).
Indicate whether each of the following statements is **True** or **False**. Question numbers correspond to learning objectives from which the questions were drawn.

1. ___ The rarity of a behavior is <u>not</u> sufficient for labelling a behavior abnormal.
2. ___ The view that abnormal behavior signifies punishment by the gods is inconsistent with the demonological model.
3. ___ The idea that abnormal behavior was rooted in diseases of the brain was first asserted by Emil Kraeplin.
4. ___ Pussin and Pinel were responsible for introducing humane treatment of abnormal behavior into asylums.
5. ___ Moral therapy assumed that normal behavior could be restored through reasoning with patients, though it was often necessary for the patients to be restrained.
6. ___ The two major factors which led to deinstitutionalization of mental hospital patients were the development of community mental health centers and the widespread use of antidepressant medications.
7. ___ The label "mentally disordered" is derived from the cognitive perspective of abnormal behavior.
8. ___ The objectives of science are description, explanation, prediction and control.
9. ___ Hypothesis formulation refers to making a precise prediction about a cause-effect relationship to be examined through research.
10. ___ In order to maximize experimental control, scientists using naturalistic observation take precautions to insure that their observation is unobtrusive.
11. ___ If a research sample is not representative of the population of interest, a threat to external validity is present.
12. ___ Correlational studies can be used to establish causation and enable prediction.
13. ___ Longitudinal studies use chronological age as a variable by selecting comparable samples of individuals differing only in age.
14. ___ Experiments are conducted to determine causal relationships.
15. ___ The single-blind method controls for the expectancies of the researcher but not the subject.

16.___ Lack of confounds is the essence of internal validity.

17.___ Quasi-experiments are useful where random assignment is not possible.

18.___ People who refuse to participate in surveys represent a major source of error in epidemiological studies.

19.___ Spontaneous improvement over time represents a serious threat to internal validity of a case study.

20.___ The multiple-line design controls for confounds by repeatedly switching from baseline to treatment and back to baseline.

Exam 2 (multiple-choice)

Select the single, best answer for each question. Question numbers correspond to learning objectives from which the questions were drawn.

1. Persistent alcohol use may be labelled abnormal primarily because it
    a. is statistically uncommon
    b. is maladaptive or self-defeating
    c. is dangerous to others
    d. violates social norms

2. Which of these is not consistent with the demonological model?
    a. exorcism
    b. persecution of mentally ill as witches
    c. excessive black bile as the cause of depression
    d. sending patients to temples dedicated to Asclepius, and providing nutrition and exercise.

3. The individual who advanced the medical model of abnormal behavior by postulating that dementia praecox and manic-depressive psychosis were due to physical problems.
    a. Emil Kraepelin
    b. Galen
    c. Edward Jenner
    d. Sigmund Freud

4. In the last half of the nineteenth century, mental hospitals in America became
   a. models of humane care of the mentally ill
   b. unnecessary due to the development of phenothiazines
   c. research laboratories for psychology
   d. little more than "human snakepits" that were all too similar to asylums

5. Benjamin Rush, the father of American psychiatry advanced the moral therapy movement by
   a. encouraging staff at his Philadelphia Hospital to treat patients with kindness and understanding.
   b. signing the Declaration of Independence.
   c. freeing mental patients from their chains.
   d. crusading across the USA against deplorable conditions in jails and almshouses.

6. Which of the following is least associated with the current exodus from mental hospitals?
   a. development of "major tranquilizers"
   b. overcrowding of mental hospitals in the first half of this century
   c. the community mental health centers act of 1963
   d. widespread adoption of the medical model of abnormal behavior

7. Contemporary model of abnormal behavior which emphasizes the need for therapists to learn to view the world from the client's perspective.
   a. medical model
   b. social learning perspective
   c. humanistic-existential perspective
   d. psychodynamic perspective

8. Which of the following is not an objective of the scientific approach to abnormal behavior?
   a. description
   b. explanation
   c. statistical analysis
   d. control

9. The statement "high levels of exercise will induce anorexia nervosa" is an example of a
   a. research question
   b. hypothesis
   c. test of a hypothesis
   d. conclusion about a hypothesis

10. Naturalistic observation
    a. provides considerable information about behavior but cannot specify why a behavior occurs.
    b. is conducted through quasi-experiments
    c. frequently employs surveys
    d. is of little value for studying abnormal behavior

11. It is necessary that a research sample be representative of the _____ of interest.
    a. behavior
    b. population
    c. experiment
    d. topic

12. A researcher found that the higher someone's intelligence the less likely it is that they will drop out of school. This finding is
    a. a positive correlation
    b. a test of a hypothesis
    c. a causal relationship
    d. a negative correlation

13. A research method which is costly and requires a time commitment that may outlive the original scientists.
    a. analogue study
    b. longitudinal study
    c. survey method
    d. epidemiological method

14. An experiment is designed to study the effect of level of anxiety on test performance. Test performance is
    a. determined by random assignment
    b. the independent variable
    c. the dependent variable
    d. a self-report measure

15. In a double-blind study
    a. subjects are unaware of which treatment they are receiving
    b. the researcher administering the treatment is unaware of which treatment is being administered
    c. both a and b are true
    d. no one knows who is given what treatment

16. The extent to which treatment effects can be accounted for by the theoretical mechanisms that are present in the independent variable is called
    a. construct validity
    b. external validity
    c. internal validity
    d. significance

17. A research method to determine causal relationships when random assignment is not possible is called a
    a. longitudinal study
    b. quasi-experiment
    c. correlational study
    d. single-blind experiment

10

18. Which of the following is <u>not</u> a source of error in epidemiological studies?
    a. inaccuracy in public health data
    b. people refusing to participate
    c. haphazard sampling
    d. confounding variables

19. Freud's study of Anna O. was a famous one.
    a. case study
    b. single-subject experiment
    c. single-blind study
    d. double-blind study

20. A single-subject research method in the form of A-B-A-B is called
    a. a longitudinal study
    b. a case study
    c. a multiple-baseline design
    d. a reversal design

TERMS AND CONCEPTS

Lesson 1
abnormal psychology (2)
unusual behavior (2)
socially unacceptable (3)
faulty perception of reality (3)
severe personal distress (4)
maladaptive behavior (4)
dangerous behavior (4)

Lesson 2
demonological model (5)
exorcism (7)
Hippocrates (6)
humors in the body (6)
medical model (7,12)
medieval view (7)
John Weyer (9)
asylums (9)
Wilhelm Griesinger (10)
Galen (7)
Dorthea Dix (11)
Emil Kraeplin (10)
Jean-Baptiste Pussin (11)
moral therapy (11)
Phillipe Pinel (11)
Benjamin Rush (11)
Louis Pasteur (10)
deinstitutionalization (12)

Lesson 3
medical model (12)
psychodynamic model (13)
learning perspective (15)
humanistic-existential perspective (16)
cognitive perspective (17)
sociocultural perspective (17)
eclectic models (17)
psychoanalysis (14)
Sigmund Freud (14-15)
behavior therapy (16)
social learning theory (16)
Rogers and Maslow (16)
Watson, Skinner and Pavlov (16)
Ellis and Beck (17)

Lesson 4
objectives of science (18)
description (18)
explanation (19)
prediction (19)
control (19)
scientific method (19)
naturalistic observation (20)
significant differences (19)
research sample (20)
population (20)
correlation (21)

negative correlation (21)
positive correlation (21)
causal relationships (21,22)
longitudinal study (21)

Lesson 5
experimental method (22)
independent variable (22)
dependent variable (22)
random assignment (22)
selection factor (22)
placebo (23)
single-blind (23)
double-blind (23)
experimental validity (24)
internal validity (24)
external validity (24)
construct validity (25)
random sampling (24)
analogue study (24)
quasi-experiment (25)
epidemiological method (26)
stratified random sampling (26)

Lesson 6
case study (27)
single-case experimental design (28)
reversal design (28)
multiple-baseline design (29)

TYING THINGS TOGETHER

1. In all likelihood, you can think of someone you know whose behavior is quite unusual. Here is your challenge: Describe this person's behavior and then analyze it in terms of the six criteria of this chapter to decide why it should or should not be labelled abnormal. [IMPORTANT: You should not use the person's real name (take a hint from Freud and the case of Anna O., which was not the patient's real name). Give the person a phony name.

2. If you have formed a study group, conduct a discussion about modern mental health care where each of you chooses to play the part of one of the historical figures from the chapter.

3. Most daily newspapers report interesting scientific findings. Unfortunately, they sometimes draw inappropriate conclusions. They are especially prone to making causal attributions from non-experimental research. Your task is to clip some interesting articles from your local paper that relate to abnormal behavior (health issues if you cannot find abnormal behavior articles) and critique them based on what you have learned about scientific methods. Try to use all of the terms and concepts from this section of your text in your critique.

4. Go to your library and find out what journals are available that focus on abnormal behavior and its treatment. Then find a recent issue for two of these journals. Look up three articles in each one to see what kind of research method it used (you will have a total of six: 2 journals X 3 articles).

ANSWERS

Lesson 1
1 b
2 f
3 a
4 g
5 c
6 e
7 d

Lesson 2
1 j
2 g
3 r
4 d
5 k
6 l
7 h
8 n
9 b
10 q
11 m
12 p

13 o
14 e
15 a
16 f
17 c
18 i

Lesson 3
1 m
2 f
3 g
4 c
5 k
6 e
7 h
8 j
9 n
10 b
11 l
12 i
13 d
14 m

Lesson 4
1 b
2 e
3 o
4 n
5 d
6 i
7 g
8 a
9 c
10 k
11 f
12 l
13 j
14 h
15 m

Lesson 5
1 m
2 n
3 e
4 h

5 i
6 q
7 b
8 j
9 d
10 l
11 k
12 o
13 f
14 a
15 g
16 p
17 c

Lesson 6
1 e
2 a
3 f
4 b
5 c
6 d

True-False answers
1 T
2 F
3 F
4 T
5 F
6 F
7 F
8 T
9 T
10 F
11 T
12 F
13 F
14 T
15 F
16 T
17 T
18 T
19 T
20 F

Multiple-Choice answers
1 b
2 c
3 a
4 d
5 a
6 d
7 c
8 c
9 b
10 a
11 b
12 d
13 b
14 c
15 c
16 a
17 b
18 d
19 a
20 d

2 Theoretical Perspectives

OVERVIEW

Chapter two expands objective 7 of the first chapter (and lesson 3 of this study guide) to chapter length. That should tell you something about the importance of the contents of this chapter. In fact, you will discover that this chapter serves as a framework for much of the rest of the text. Presentation of various behavior disorders in the rest of the text will be organized around the perspectives presented in this chapter. More depth of learning in this chapter will pay you considerable benefit later in the course. The chapter is organized around six contemporary perspectives. Each perspective is explained in detail, and then critically evaluated (strengths and weaknesses). Lessons in this chapter generally correspond to the major sections of the chapter, except that sociocultural perspective was combined with humanistic-existential perspective into a single lesson, due to the relative length of material.

The psychodynamic perspective focuses on unconscious, internal psychological conflict as the critical determinant of abnormal behavior. The learning perspective contrasts sharply with this view. Much of the focus is on factors external to the individual as determinants of behavior. These are the factors that influence learning processes. Cognitive perspectives focus on the role of cognitions (mental processes including perception, memory, thoughts, problem solving) as determinants of abnormal behavior. The humanistic-existential perspective places considerable emphasis on personal freedom and choices we make in the quest for purpose and meaning in our lives. The sociocultural perspective focuses on social and cultural factors as explanations for abnormal behavior. The brevity of this section reflects the scope of this area, but not its impact on abnormal psychology. The biological perspective focuses on abnormal behavior with known biological determinants. A focused review of the major concepts of behavioral neural science provides key background information for understanding the presentations of these disorders in later chapters.

CHAPTER OUTLINE, LESSONS & LEARNING OBJECTIVES

Lesson 1. Psychodynamic perspectives. (36-46)
PSYCHODYNAMIC PERSPECTIVES. (36-46)
1. Identify and briefly describe the basic tenants of Sigmund Freud's psychodynamic theory.
2. Compare and contrast more recent psychodynamic theories to the views of Freud.
3. Critically evaluate psychodynamic theories.

Lesson 2. Learning perspectives. (46-55)
LEARNING PERSPECTIVES. (46-55)
4. Understand the viewpoint of behaviorism and describe the principles of conditioning.
5. Identify and describe social learning theory and the situational and personal variables that influence behavior.
6. Critically evaluate learning theories.

Lesson 3. Cognitive perspectives. (55-58)
COGNITIVE PERSPECTIVES. (55-58)
7. Describe the information processing approach and the theoretical contributions of George Kelley, Albert Ellis and Aaron Beck.
8. Critically evaluate cognitive theories.

Lesson 4. Humanistic-existential and sociocultural perspectives. (58-65)
9. Describe the basic tenants of humanistic and existential philosophies.
10. Summarize the views of Viktor Frankl, Abraham Maslow and Carl Rogers.
11. Critically evaluate humanistic-existential theories.
SOCIOCULTURAL PERSPECTIVES. (63-65)
12. Describe the sociocultural views of abnormal behavior.
13. Critically evaluate the sociocultural perspectives.

Lesson 5. Biological perspectives. (65-74)
BIOLOGICAL PERSPECTIVES. (65-74)
14. Describe the basic structure and function of the nervous system; be able to describe the means by which neurons communicate with each other.
15. Identify the basic structures of the brain and their functions.
16. Describe the functions of the endocrine system and the effects of hormones on human behavior.
17. Explain how kinship studies suggest roles for genetic factors as determinants of abnormal behavior.
18. Critically evaluate theories concerning the relationships between biological structures and processes and abnormal behavior.

Mastering Lesson 1. Psychodynamic perspectives. (36-46)

Since the psychoanalytic theory of Sigmund Freud is both the origin and central focus of the psychodynamic perspective, it forms much of the basis for this lesson. The best way to approach learning psychoanalytic theory is to make "passes" through the material. First learn the terminology and appropriate groupings [learning the associations represented by the double ended arrows, for instance: mental geography <--> conscious, preconscious and unconscious; personality structures <--> id, ego and superego]. As you learn terminology, associate things with how they work [e.g., ego <--> reality principle]. The "second pass" is the real key to understanding. Do not cheat yourself by thinking, "I know this stuff really well, so I can skip the second pass." Go through the material a second time and relate things from different groupings together. Ask yourself things like, "What is the mental geography or consciousness level of anal fixations? How are the personality structures conflicting in the development of the Oedipus conflict?" This second pass will not be easy, but it will give you valuable practice using the new vocabulary and help you tie all of the concepts into a coherent theoretical view at the same time.

This lesson also includes contributions of several individuals who were influenced by psychoanalytic theory. Here you should learn to associate the prominent individuals with their points of departure--where they differed from Freud. All of the lessons in this chapter end with an evaluation objective. In this lesson, you will learn to identify the major strengths and shortcomings of the psychoanalytic perspective as a theoretical model and as it influenced the broader field of abnormal psychology.

Match the following terms and concepts with the correct definition or description or explanation.

1. __ Alfred Adler
2. __ anal
3. __ Carl Jung
4. __ collective unconscious
5. __ defense mechanisms
6. __ ego
7. __ ego psychology
8. __ Erik Erikson
9. __ genital
10. __ geography of the mind
11. __ id
12. __ latency
13. __ neurotic anxiety
14. __ oral
15. __ personality structures
16. __ phallic
17. __ psychic determinism
18. __ psychosexual stages
19. __ superego

a. id, ego and superego
b. unconscious, conscious and preconscious
c. sexual impulses are silent
d. accumulated experience of mankind
e. neo-freudian who thought our unconscious experience included archetypes
f. neo-freudian who substituted inferiority complex for the sexual motivation of Freud
g. oral, anal, phallic, latency and genital
h. behavior determined by interaction of mental processes
i. psychic structure governed by the moral principle
j. sucking and biting are sources of sexual stimulation
k. ego senses that unacceptable impulses of id might become conscious
l. recent psychodynamic models replacing emphasis on sexual instinct with emphasis on the self
m. dominated by sexual feelings towards opposite sex
n. psychic structure which follows the pleasure principle
o. psychic structure governed by the reality principle
p. emphasized the influence of children's social relations on ego development
q. elimination as focus of sexual stimulation
r. unconscious ego processes that protect us from unpleasant cognitions
s. phallic region as primary erogenous zone

Mastering Lesson 2. Learning perspectives. (46-55)

While the psychodynamic perspective looks within the individual for the source of abnormal behavior, the learning perspective looks for causal factors primarily outside of the individual. These factors are the environmental influences that shape and maintain our behavior. The chapter divides the learning perspective into behaviorism and social learning theory; behaviorism is presented first with a brief explanation of the principles of classical and operant conditioning.

Mastery of this objective involves learning some principles of classical conditioning, operant conditioning and social learning theory. Then you will learn how these principles are applied to abnormal behavior. Finally, you will understand the major strengths and criticisms of the learning perspective of abnormal behavior.

Match the following terms and concepts with the correct definition or description or explanation.

1. __ classical conditioning
2. __ conditioned response
3. __ conditioned stimulus
4. __ extinction
5. __ negative reinforcers
6. __ observational learning
7. __ operant conditioning
8. __ person variables
9. __ positive reinforcer
10. __ primary reinforcers
11. __ punishment
12. __ secondary reinforcers
13. __ self-efficacy expectations
14. __ social learning theory
15. __ spontaneous recovery
16. __ unconditioned response
17. __ unconditioned stimulus

a. learning approaches of Albert Bandura, Walter Mischel and Julian Rotter

b. response which is elicited by a CS as a result of CS-US pairing

c. factors within an individual which must be considered in explaining behavior

d. suppressing behavior by delivery of painful, aversive events

e. recurrence of an extinguished CR which results from passage of time

f. response elicited by a stimulus without prior learning

g. stimulus which elicits a specific response without learning

h. conditioning in which responses are emitted because of their consequences

i. elimination of a CR by repeated presentation of the CS alone

j. acquisition of new behaviors by observing the performance of others

k. reinforcers that must be paired with primary reinforcers to be effective

l. stimulus which elicits a response as a result of pairing with a US

m. individual's beliefs about the likelihood of personal success at a task

n. events presented after a behavior that increase the behavior

o. events removed after a behavior that decrease the behavior

p. a stimulus paired with another stimulus comes to elicit a new response

q. reinforcers which do not require prior experience to work

Mastering Lesson 3. Cognitive perspectives. (55-58)

This lesson presents four cognitive perspectives. The first, information processing, uses the computer as a metaphor. It is the most recent development paralleling access to computing in our society. The other three are more established models developed by George Kelly, Albert Ellis, and Aaron Beck. In mastering this lesson you will learn the views of each model. Pay attention to the kinds of cognitions each selects to focus on, how these cognitions are related to abnormal behavior and the kinds of treatment strategies they suggest.

Match the following terms and concepts with the correct definition or description or explanation.

1. __ Aaron Beck
2. __ absolutist thinking
3. __ Albert Ellis
4. __ cognition
5. __ cognitive therapy
6. __ George Kelly
7. __ information processing
8. __ magnification
9. __ overgeneralization
10. __ personal constructs
11. __ rational-emotive therapy
12. __ selective abstraction

a. drawing broad conclusions from a few isolated failures
b. developed cognitive therapy to help clients identify and correct cognitive errors
c. psychological dimensions by which we categorize ourselves, others and our experiences
d. developed model based on the way people construe events
e. developer of rational-emotive therapy
f. based on irrational beliefs resulting in maladaptive behavior
g. focusing on personal flaws while ignoring competencies
h. model that attempts to correct four basic types of cognitive errors
i. it's total success or nothing
j. blowing unfortunate events out of proportion
k. model using concepts like input, processing, storage and retrieval
l. a word for mental processes

Lesson 4. Humanistic-existential and sociocultural perspectives. (58-65)

The humanistic-existential perspective is rooted in the philosophical school of existentialism. The lesson begins with a brief statement of this philosophical position. The humanistic positions of Viktor Frankl, Abraham Maslow and Carl Rogers are also presented. Learn not only how each is unique, but also what they have in common that gets them grouped into the humanistic-existential perspective.

Since it is very brief, we have decided to include the sociocultural perspective in this lesson. In the search for causation, the sociocultural perspective has looked to the ills of society for a focus. The description of Thomas Szasz's position on labeling abnormal behavior as illness has had a major impact on the field of abnormal psychology.

Match the following terms and concepts with the correct definition or description or explanation.

1. __ Abraham Maslow
2. __ Carl Rogers
3. __ existentialism
4. __ hierarchy of needs
5. __ humanism
6. __ logotherapy
7. __ R. D. Laing
8. __ self-actualization
9. __ self-theory
10. __ Thomas Szasz
11. __ unconditional positive regard
12. __ Viktor Frankl

a. biological, safety, love and belongingness, esteem and self-actualization
b. focuses on self as the executive of personality
c. survivor of Nazi concentration camps and developer of logotherapy
d. argued that people have growth-oriented needs for self-actualization
e. argued that mental illness is a myth used to subjugate people
f. believes that double messages and confused social mores stifle adaptive, productive action
g. a therapy based on helping people find ways of talking about and organizing their lives
h. taking risks in order to reach our maximum potentials
i. accepting value of others regardless of the worth of their behavior at a moment in time
j. philosophy concerned with questions of our existence
k. minister-turned-psychologist who developed self-theory
l. emerged as reaction to the rat race, placed emphasis on the meaning of life

Mastering Lesson 5. Biological perspectives. (65-74)

The biological perspective is a bit of a departure from the information presented in objective 7 (lesson 3) of chapter one. This lesson will focus on identified physiological/biological problems associated with abnormal behavior. In order to fully appreciate this material, and related information in later chapters, it is essential to have a bit of background information about the nervous system and how it works. The textbook begins with just such an overview. As you go through the sections that comprise this lesson, try to associate structures (brain areas, parts of neurons, etc) with their functions. Practice these associations in both directions (structure --> function and function --> structure), as both kinds of questions are readily written for examinations. Behavioral genetics are also included in this section, because some forms of abnormal behavior are believed to be inherited. Here, the best approach is to learn the terminology and try to understand the goals of behavioral genetics and how the methods presented in this section contribute to reaching these goals.

Match the following terms and concepts with the correct definition or description or explanation.

1. __ autonomic nervous system
2. __ axon
3. __ axon terminals
4. __ catecholamines
5. __ central nervous system
6. __ cerebellum
7. __ dendrites
8. __ endocrine system
9. __ genotype
10. __ hypothalamus
11. __ limbic system
12. __ medulla
13. __ neuron
14. __ neurotransmitters
15. __ norepinephrine
16. __ phenotype
17. __ reticular activating system
18. __ serotonin
19. __ synapse
20. __ thalamus

a. adrenalin and noradrenalin
b. divided into sympathetic and parasympathetic branches
c. brain and spinal cord
d. long, trunk-like projection from cell body
e. junction between two neurons
f. the genetic makeup of an individual
g. receive messages from other neurons
h. physical expression of our genetic makeup
i. the ductless glands, taken together
j. basic unit of the nervous system
k. relays sensory information to cerebral cortex
l. part of brain involved in attention and arousal
m. small branches where axons end that contain knobs
n. chemicals which allow neural messages to cross synapse
o. group of structures involved in memory, hunger, sex, aggression
p. a neurotransmitter involved in learning and memory
q. neurotransmitter linked to anxiety, insomnia and mood disorders
r. brain structure that controls homeostatic regulation, motivation
s. brain structure involved in balance and motor control
t. area of brainstem that controls heart rate and respiration

PRACTICE EXAMS

Exam 1. (true-false).

Indicate whether each of the following statements is **True** or **False**. Question numbers correspond to learning objectives from which the questions were drawn.

1. __ Anal fixations deriving from conflicts over toilet training can lead to development of anal-retentive traits which include carelessness and messiness.
2. __ Alfred Adler differed from Freud by attributing more importance to children's social relationships than to unconscious processes.
3. __ Though controversial, Freud's psychanalytic theory was the first to recognize that defense processes could distort a person's perceptions of their feelings, needs and desires.
4. __ You may come to fear the dentist's office after a painful experience there. In classical conditioning this fear would be called a conditioned stimulus.
5. __ The person variables emphasized in social learning theory include expectancies, competencies, plans and encoding strategies.

6. __ Critics of social learning theory contend that it cannot explain the richness of human behavior, and that it is overly mechanistic.

7. __ Personal constructs are valuable because they help us to interpret the world around us and anticipate events.

8. __ Cognitive approaches to therapy focus on the present, while psychodynamic therapies focus on the past.

9. __ Humanism developed out of complaints of alienation that resulted from industrialization.

10. __ Maslow's hierarchy of needs includes biological, love/belonging, safety, esteem, power and self-actualization.

11. __ Humanistic-existential theories have been criticized because they focus on conscious experience which is not publicly observable.

12. __ R. D. Laing argued that double messages lead to abnormal behavior by preventing us from experiencing unconditional positive regard.

13. __ Epidemiological evidence has supported sociocultural perspectives by showing that lower socioeconomic classes were more likely to be institutionalized for abnormal behavior, while upper classes were more likely to be encouraged to seek outpatient care.

14. __ Transmission of neural messages across the synapse is accomplished by minute electrical charges.

15. __ Damage to the cerebellum results in loss of motor coordination.

16. __ Catecholamines, released by the adrenal medulla, are responsible for regulation of basal metabolic rate.

17. __ In order to determine whether a pattern of abnormal behavior has a genetic basis, researchers first isolate a suspected genotype and then study how that genotype is distributed in family members.

18. __ While biological perspectives have resulted in identification of some disorders with a biological basis and hold much promise for the future, they have contributed little that is useful in the treatment of abnormal behavior.

Exam 2 (multiple-choice)

Select the single, best answer for each question. Question numbers correspond to learning objectives from which the questions were drawn.

1. Freud's structures of personality are
   a. pleasure, reality and moral
   b. id, ego and superego
   c. unconscious, conscious and preconscious
   d. oral, anal, phallic latent and genital

2. Freud is to Jung as
   a. unconscious conflict is to archetype
   b. ego is to inferiority complex
   c. analytical psychology is to psychoanalytic theory
   d. psychoanalytic theory is to individual psychology

3. Which of the following ideas does not represent a major contribution of psychodynamic theory?
   a. defense mechanisms can distort our perceptions
   b. behavior can be motivated by hidden drives and impulses
   c. childhood experiences play a critical role in shaping abnormal behavior
   d. people have strong needs to reach their ego ideals

4. The learning perspective argues that abnormal behavior results from things like
   a. double messages
   b. acting on irrational beliefs
   c. inappropriate or inadequate reinforcement
   d. unconscious conflict among learning experiences

5. In contrast to behaviorism, social learning theory emphasizes the importance of
   a. conditioned stimuli as sources of fear
   b. confronting irrational beliefs
   c. goal setting and self-rewards
   d. consistent application of punishment

6. The major contributions of the learning perspective include
   a. incorporating both environmental and unconscious variables into the search for causal relations in abnormal behavior
   b. emphasis on observable behavior and environmental stimuli
   c. their emphasis on the critical learning experiences which occur during the oral and anal stages of development
   d. a methodology for the experimental study of the collective unconscious

7. Which of the following is not one of Ellis's irrational beliefs?
   a. you must be completely competent in everything you do
   b. happiness will come to you without effort on your part
   c. you require continuous love and approval from those who are important to you
   d. your personal perceptions of the world are all that matters

8. Which of the following evaluative statements best applies to the cognitive perspective?
   a. cognitive theorists have focused on anxiety and depression, but it is unclear whether distorted thinking is a cause or an effect of depression
   b. cognitive models have not led to effective therapies
   c. cognitive models are applicable to broad ranges of abnormal behavior
   d. anal-expressive traits are readily explained by cognitive models while anal-retentive traits are not

9. Existentialism is a philosophical school concerned with the larger questions of existence that confront us as we come to terms with
   a. being in the world and mortality
   b. irrational beliefs and unconscious conflict
   c. reality
   d. competing in the "rat race"

10. Which of the following is <u>not</u> a humanistic-existential theorist?
    a. Abraham Maslow
    b. Alfred Adler
    c. Viktor Frankl
    d. Carl Rogers

11. A major problem with Maslow's concept of self-actualization is that it
    a. yields circular explanations of behavior
    b. does not apply to nonhumans
    c. is easily measured but not predicted
    d. has been repeatedly disproved

12. Which of the following is <u>not</u> an argument against mental illness posed by the sociocultural perspective?
    a. mental illness stigmatizes individuals who display deviant behavior
    b. labels of mental illness further stigmatize the individual
    c. abnormal behavior is the problem rather than a symptom of underlying illness
    d. once applied to an individual, the mental illness label is difficult to get rid of

13. The sociocultural writings of Szasz
    a. have led to development of therapeutic approaches
    b. apply primarily to labels arising out of the psychodynamic perspective
    c. have been ignored by mental health workers
    d. have been somewhat outmoded due to deinstitutionalization

14. The structure of a neuron which propagates messages over long distances is called
    a. a synapse
    b. a dendrite
    c. an axon
    d. a soma

15. Which of the following brain structures is associated with its function?
    a. medulla--balance, coordination
    b. sympathetic nervous system--eating
    c. hypothalamus--arousal and sleep
    d. thalamus--sensory relay

16. Dizziness, lack of energy and trembling are symptoms of
    a. hypoglycemia
    b. hyperglycemia
    c. hyperthyroidism
    d. anabolic steroid use

17. The diathesis-stress model of genetic-environment interaction suggests that
    a. genotypic vulnerability combined with environmental stress yields abnormal behavior
    b. phenotypic vulnerability plus inappropriate learning yields abnormal behavior
    c. intrauterine, prenatal stress alters genotype to produce vulnerability
    d. genotypic vulnerability produces stress which yields abnormal behavior that is inappropriate to the environment

18. Which of the following is not a major limitation to twin studies?
    a. lack of access to adoption records
    b. MZ twins receiving greater encouragement to act alike
    c. finding MZ twins who were separated at birth
    d. the difficulty in finding MZ twins living in comparable socioeconomic classes to DZ twins

TERMS AND CONCEPTS

Lesson 1
Alfred Adler (43)
anal stage(40)
Carl Jung (42)
collective unconscious (42)
defense mechanisms (38)
ego (37)
ego psychology (43)
Electra complex (41)
Erik Erikson (43)
genital stage(42)
geography of the mind (37)
id (37)
latency stage (42)
neurotic anxiety (39)
Oedipus complex (41)
oral stage (40)
personality structures (37)
phallic stage(41)
psychic determinism (36)
psychosexual stages (40)
superego (37)

Lesson 2
classical conditioning (47)
conditioned response (48)
conditioned stimulus (47)
extinction (48)
negative reinforcers (49)
observational learning (51)
operant conditioning (49)
person variables (51)
positive reinforcer (49)

primary reinforcers (49)
punishment (50)
secondary reinforcers (50)
self-efficacy expectations (52)
social learning theory (50)
spontaneous recovery (48)
unconditioned response (47)
unconditioned stimulus (47)

Lesson 3
Aaron Beck (57)
absolutist thinking (57)
Albert Ellis (56)
cognition (55)
cognitive therapy (57)
George Kelly (55)
information processing (55)
magnification (57)
overgeneralization (57)
personal constructs (56)
rational-emotive therapy (56)
selective abstraction (57)

Lesson 4
Abraham Maslow (60)
Carl Rogers (61)
existentialism (58)
hierarchy of needs (61)
humanism (58)
logotherapy (59)

R. D. Laing (64)
self-actualization (60)
self-theory (61)
Thomas Szasz (63)
unconditional positive regard (62)
Viktor Frankl (59)

Lesson 5
autonomic nervous system (68)
axon (65)
axon terminals (65)
catecholamines (70)
central nervous system (65)
cerebellum (67)
dendrites (65)
endocrine system (69)
genotype (71)
hypothalamus (67)
limbic system (68)
medulla (67)
neuron (65)
neurotransmitters (65)
norepinephrine (65)
phenotype (71)
reticular activating system (67)
serotonin (65)
synapse (65)
thalamus (67)

TYING THINGS TOGETHER

1. At first glance, one might assume that abnormal behavior with known organic causes are only treatable by medical means; if there is no medical treatment available, then the disorder is not treatable. That is not necessarily true. Your challenge is to choose one of the perspectives in this chapter and decide what you would do to treat a patient suffering from Alzheimer's disease. Can you think of some things to do to allow this patient to function better?

2. In chapter one, a seventh perspective was mentioned. The eclectic view combined the best ideas of the other perspectives. Now that you know more about the six perspectives, write down the list of things you would include in your own eclectic view.

ANSWERS

Lesson 1
1 f
2 q
3 e
4 d
5 r
6 o
7 l
8 p
9 m
10 b
11 n
12 c
13 k
14 j
15 a
16 s
17 h
18 g
19 i

Lesson 2
1 p
2 b
3 l
4 i
5 o
6 j
7 h
8 c
9 n
10 q
11 d
12 k
13 m
14 a
15 e
16 f
17 g

Lesson 3
1 b
2 i
3 e
4 l
5 h
6 d
7 k
8 j
9 a
10 c
11 f
12 g

Lesson 4
1 d
2 k
3 j
4 a
5 l
6 g
7 f
8 h
9 b
10 e
11 i
12 c

Lesson 5

1 b
2 d
3 m
4 a
5 c

6 s
7 g
8 i
9 f
10 r
11 o
12 t
13 j
14 n
15 p
16 h
17 l
18 q
19 e
20 k

True-False answers
1 F
2 F
3 T
4 F
5 T
6 F
7 T
8 T
9 T
10 F
11 T
12 F
13 T
14 F
15 T
16 F
17 F
18 F

Multiple-Choice answers
1 b
2 a
3 d
4 c
5 c
6 b
7 d
8 a
9 b
10 b
11 a
12 c
13 d
14 c
15 d
16 a
17 a
18 d

3 Classification and Assessment of Abnormal Behavior

OVERVIEW

While the previous chapters have provided a general perspective on abnormal behavior and research methods, this chapter moves closer to abnormal behavior, looking not so much at the larger picture, but at the methods we use to assess and classify abnormal behavior. The DSM-III-R classification system is presented first. It represents a framework used by the medical and psychological communities. Major portions of this textbook are organized around DSM-III-R groupings of disorders.

After reviewing issues of reliability and validity as they apply to psychological tests, the chapter focuses on three major types of tests, intelligence tests, personality tests and neuropsychological assessment instruments. The final sections of the chapter present other assessment methods in the behavioral and cognitive areas as well as some emerging technology in direct physiological measurement and medical imaging. You should view all of these assessment methods as a relatively comprehensive tool kit for assessing abnormal behavior. Generally, information from several of these methods is gathered and assembled before an individual is classified in the DSM-III-R system.

CHAPTER OUTLINE, LESSONS & LEARNING OBJECTIVES

Lesson 1. Introduction to DSM-III-R. (79-86)
CLASSIFICATION OF ABNORMAL BEHAVIOR. (79-86)
1. Understand the historical origins of modern diagnostic systems.
2. Define the concept of "mental disorders" in the DSM-III-R system and describe its relation to the medical model.
3. Describe the features of the DSM-III-R system.
4. Explain the multiaxial features of DSM-III-R
5. Describe the strengths and weaknesses of DSM-III-R

Lesson 2. Reliability and validity of assessment methods. (86-88)
CHARACTERISTICS OF METHODS OF ASSESSMENT. (86-88)
6. Understand reliability and the three approaches to demonstrating reliability of assessment methods.
7. Understand validity and the three approaches to demonstrating validity of assessment methods.

Lesson 3. Clinical interviewing. (88-93)

THE CLINICAL INTERVIEW. (88-93)

8. Describe what is meant by the structured interview.
9. Describe the elements of the mental status examination.
10. Summarize the major aspects of effective interviewing.
11. Describe the use of standardized interview techniques.

Lesson 4. Psychological tests for assessment of intelligence, personality and neurological function. (93-106)

PSYCHOLOGICAL TESTS. (93-95)

12. Understand the nature and value of psychological tests.

INTELLIGENCE TESTS. (95-97)

13. Summarize the history and features of the Stanford-Binet.
14. Discuss the features of the Wechsler scales.

PERSONALITY TESTS. (97-104)

15. Distinguish between self-report and projective personality assessment techniques.
16. Discuss the history, features, reliability and validity of personality tests, focusing on the MMPI, Rorschach and TAT.

NEUROPSYCHOLOGICAL ASSESSMENT. (104-106)

17. Describe the use of psychological tests in the assessment of neuropsychological functioning.

Lesson 5. Behavioral assessment, cognitive assessment and physiological measurement. (106-114)

BEHAVIORAL ASSESSMENT (106-110)

18. Summarize the advantages and limitations to behavioral assessment.
19. Describe the behavioral assessment techniques of the behavioral interview, self-monitoring, use of contrived measures, direct observation and behavioral rating scales.

COGNITIVE ASSESSMENT (110-111)

20. Discuss the use of thought diaries and questionnaires that assess automatic thoughts and dysfunctional attitudes.

PHYSIOLOGICAL MEASUREMENT (111-114)

21. Describe the relationships between emotional states and physiological measurement.
22. Describe contemporary imaging techniques.

Mastering Lesson 1. Introduction to DSM-III-R. (79-86)

DSM stands for Diagnostic and Statistical Manual; the most recent version is a revision to the third edition, hence the III-R. In this lesson, you will understand the historical background of the DSM system, be able to describe its features and explain how it is used. You will also learn its strengths and weaknesses. The matching exercise below is intended to help you develop fluency with some of the key terms and concepts of DSM-III-R.

Match the following terms and concepts with the correct definition or description or explanation.

1. __ breadth of coverage
2. __ clinical syndromes
3. __ developmental disorders
4. __ DSM-III-R features
5. __ global assessment of functioning
6. __ multiaxial
7. __ personality disorders
8. __ physical conditions and disorders
9. __ reliability of DSM-III
10. __ severity of psychosocial stressors
11. __ validity of DSM-III

a. DSM-III had fewer cases classified as "other" at the expense of purity
b. DSM-III-R uses five dimensions called axes
c. multiaxial system that uses specific criteria, groups categories by shared clinical features
d. part of Axis II which includes antisocial personality disorder
e. part of Axis II, includes mental retardation
f. Axis V of DSM-III-R, rates highest two months of past year and current levels
g. Superior to DSM-II, but still low on axis II and IV
h. Axis IV of DSM-III-R, rates severity of stressful events in past year
i. Axis III of DSM-III-R, conditions that may affect functioning or response to treatment
j. Axis I of DSM-III-R, is the pattern of distressing, abnormal behavior
k. appears to predict response to treatment; generally difficult to assess

Mastering Lesson 2. Reliability and validity of assessment methods. (86-88)

Whenever assessment or measurement is mentioned, one should not take for granted that the measurement is accurate or that the measurement corresponds well to the concept being measured. These are the issues of reliability and validity. Before your text can meaningfully discuss various assessment methods, it is expedient to review these formal concepts.

Match the following terms and concepts with the correct definition or description or explanation.

1. __ coefficient alpha
2. __ concurrent validity
3. __ construct validity
4. __ content validity
5. __ criterion validity
6. __ internal consistency
7. __ interrater reliability
8. __ predictive validity
9. __ reliability
10. __ temporal stability
11. __ validity

a. correlations among items in a test
b. consistency of measurement
c. a measure of internal consistency
d. retesting yields similar results
e. does an assessment device predict future behavior
f. level of agreement between two or more judges
g. relationship of assessment responses to an external standard
h. relation of test content to underlying theory
i. measurements correspond to what they are intended to assess
j. extent to which an assessment device predicts scores on a second measuring device
k. a representative sample of behaviors associated with a construct are included

Mastering Lesson 3. Clinical interviewing. (88-93)

The clinical interview is a key assessment tool. It is the most widely used assessment technique. Usually it is the first interpersonal relationship between client and therapist, therefore it is critical for the therapist to have good interviewing skills. In this lesson you will learn about the various types of interviews and the key skills that go into the clinical interview. The matching section below will help you build fluency using the terminology of interviewing techniques.

Match the following terms and concepts with the correct definition or description or explanation.

1. __ affect
2. __ appearance
3. __ behavioral observations
4. __ clarification
5. __ insight
6. __ intake interview
7. __ intelligence
8. __ memory
9. __ mental status examination
10. __ orientation
11. __ paraphrasing
12. __ perceptual processes
13. __ presenting problem
14. __ rapport
15. __ reflection
16. __ sensorium
17. __ structured interview
18. __ summarization
19. __ thought process

a. recent and remote are categories
b. judgment of the appropriateness of grooming and attire
c. emotion client attaches to objects and ideas
d. feelings of trust between therapist and client
e. includes verbal and nonverbal behavior, manner of speech
f. complaint that leads client to seek therapy
g. client's form and content of thought
h. initial interview to learn about client's presenting problem and history
i. interviewing technique in which the interviewer rephrases the content of client's message
j. interviewing technique in which client is asked to explain his or her answers
k. judgments about client's focusing of attention and capacity for concentration
l. interviewing technique of rephrasing emotional content of client's message
m. a standard series of questions are asked to obtain clinically useful information
n. based on observations of client's behavior and questioning of cognitive functions
o. extent to which client understands and recognizes his or her problem
p. interviewing technique of tying together client's key issues or themes
q. judgments about client's understanding of who he or she is, when it is
r. extent to which client interprets and responds appropriately to sensory information
s. judgment based on client's general knowledge and ability to express ideas clearly

Mastering Lesson 4. Psychological tests for assessment of intelligence, personality and neurological function. (93-106)

This lesson serves to introduce the concept of psychological tests. The chapter focuses on three major clinical uses of tests: the assessment of intelligence, personality and neuropsychological functioning. One could view a psychological test as a highly structured situation in which to obtain a sample of behavior. In mastering this lesson, pay attention to the things that set psychological tests apart from interview techniques. Ask what kinds of information the results of a particular test provide, and how the test manages to get from the sample of behavior it obtains to those results.

Issues of reliability and validity of psychological tests are of considerable importance. If it has been awhile since you completed lesson two on reliability and validity, it would be a great idea to review that lesson before proceeding. The matching section that follows will help you develop the technical vocabulary you need to master this objective.

Match the following terms and concepts with the correct definition or description or explanation.

1. ___ contrasted groups approach
2. ___ deviation IQ
3. ___ Hermann Rorschach
4. ___ intelligence
5. ___ IQ
6. ___ Louis Terman
7. ___ MMPI
8. ___ neuropsychological assessment
9. ___ Personality Tests
10. ___ projective tests
11. ___ psychological tests
12. ___ self-report
13. ___ self-report symptom questionnaires
14. ___ standard scores
15. ___ Stanford-Binet Intelligence Scale
16. ___ Thematic Apperception Test
17. ___ validity scales
18. ___ Wechsler Scales

a. BDI and HSCL are economical examples that have high reliability
b. self-report and projective are its major types
c. the capacity to understand the world and cope with its challenges
d. establishes concurrent validity of the MMPI
e. an intelligence test based on the concepts of mental age and chronological age
f. an IQ measure based on deviation from norms of an age group
g. an objective personality test scored based on answers given by clinical and normal groups
h. objective personality tests that use forced-choice format
i. developed projective test using inkblots as stimuli
j. the ratio of mental age to chronological age multiplied by 100
k. clients' responses to ambiguous stimuli include their own needs, drives and motives
l. MMPI scales that detect clients trying to "fake good" or "fake bad"
m. highly structured assessment devices with norms from large numbers of individuals
n. projective test developed by Murray that uses pictures of ambiguous scenes
o. adapted the Binet-Simon test for use with American Children
p. In the MMPI, they have a mean of 50 and standard deviation of 10
q. uses verbal and performance subtests
r. Bender Visual Motor Gestalt, Halstead-Reitan and Luria Nebraska are examples

33

Mastering Lesson 5.   Behavioral assessment, cognitive assessment and physiological measurement. (106-114).

The topics grouped together in this lesson might appear to be a potpourri of things, but in fact that is not the case. They all have one thing in common. They look to the environment for the source of abnormal behavior. They examine the (antecedent) situation in which the behavior occurs, the behavior itself and the consequences of the behavior which tend to maintain it. The assumption is that abnormal behavior is specific to the situation in which it occurs and is maintained by its consequences. Cognitions are viewed as a special kind of behavior (observable only by the individual) that has the same kinds of lawful relationships to antecedents and consequences.

This is a very different focus from that of psychological tests. The use of tests assumes that causes are within the individual. Thus tests attempt to measure enduring characteristics of the individual (intelligence, personality traits) that are responsible for abnormal behavior across a wide variety of situations.

In mastering this objective, think of behavioral assessment as having "A-B-Cs. These techniques all try to assess the Antecedents, Behaviors (including cognitions), and Consequences. You need to learn how each of the different techniques in this lesson go about assessing these A-B-Cs.

The final objectives focus on measurement of brain function. They share the emphasis direct assessment, but an A-B-Cs analysis is not an appropriate way to organize your knowledge here. Rather you should try to associate different techniques with what they are actually measuring. The matching section that follows will help you add the vocabulary of behavioral and cognitive assessment to your repertoire of knowledge and skill.

Match the following terms and concepts with the correct definition or description or explanation.

1. __	analogue measures	a.	noninvasive measurement of electrical activity of brain
2. __	BEAM		
3. __	behavioral assessment	b.	behavior change resulting from being observed
4. __	behavioral interview	c.	commonly uses a thought diary
5. __	behavioral rating scale	d.	measures tension by assessing electrical activity in muscle
6. __	CAT scan		
7. __	cognitive assessment	e.	observations made in role-playing situations
8. __	direct observation	f.	observation of behavior in the normal environment
9. __	electrodermal response	g.	checklist of behaviors that provides information about frequency and intensity
10.__	electroencephalograph		
11.__	electromyograph	h.	map of brain obtained by computer analysis of brain wave patterns
12.__	functional analysis		
13.__	NMR	i.	finding relationship of behavior to its antecedents and consequences
14.__	PET scan		
15.__	reactivity	j.	measures changes in skin conductivity to determine anxiety level
16.__	self-monitoring		

k. view of brain activity produced by computer analysis of glucose radioisotope

l. individual records behavior as it occurs using diary or wrist counter

m. view of brain produced by computer analysis of reflected radio waves

n. asking questions about behavior and its relationship to situational factors

o. treats behaviors as resulting from environmental situation in which they occur

p. view of brain produced by computerized analysis of x-rays

PRACTICE EXAMS

Exam 1. (true-false).
Indicate whether each of the following statements is True or False. Question numbers correspond to learning objectives from which the questions were drawn.

1. __ DSM-III-R is a current system of classification based on the medical model.
2. __ DSM-III-R treats abnormal behavior as symptoms of underlying pathology.
3. __ The multi-axial diagnostic system encourages psychologists to base their diagnosis on a single, most prominent symptom.
4. __ An unwanted pregnancy would be listed on axis IV of DSM-III-R.
5. __ DSM-III-R suffers from focusing on disorders people have rather than what these people can do in specific kinds of situations.
6. __ An individual would repeatedly administer the same test to the same individual in order to determine its coefficient alpha.
7. __ One type of content validity is called face validity.
8. __ Intake interviews use the mental status examination.

9. __ The mental status exam requires the interviewer to make judgments based on the client's verbal and nonverbal behavior about various aspects of the client's cognitive functioning.

10. __ Effective interviewing techniques include clarification, summarization, reflection and paraphrasing.

11. __ Reliability of diagnostic judgments based on interviews is not affected by standardization.

12. __ Psychological tests are readily quantified which insures high reliability and validity.

13. __ The Stanford-Binet has abandoned the intelligence quotient in favor of a deviation IQ measure.

14. __ The Wechsler scales allow computation of verbal and performance IQs.

15. __ Projective tests of personality utilize a forced-choice format.

16. __ The reliability of projective tests tend to be higher than reliability of self-report personality measures.

17. __ Response patterns on the Luria-Nebraska Test Battery reveal skill deficits that suggest specific sites of brain damage.

18. __ A major limitation to behavioral assessment is reactivity which has been shown to permanently bias results of behavioral observations.

19. __ The behavioral approach task is an example of a contrived measure.

20. __ Thought diaries have been shown to assess cognitions with a high degree of reliability.

21. __ Anxiety is associated with arousal of the sympathetic nervous system which is measured as decreased skin conductivity.

22. __ In the PET scan, the patient is placed in a strong magnetic field and scanned with a narrow band of x-rays.

Exam 2 (multiple-choice)

Select the single, best answer for each question. Question numbers correspond to learning objectives from which the questions were drawn.

1. The DSM classification system is an outgrowth of the work of
   a. B. F. Skinner
   b. Emil Kraepelin
   c. Aristotle
   d. Sigmund Freud

2. A mental disorder (in DSM-III-R) requires
   a. statistically uncommon behavior
   b. an expected response to a stressful event
   c. emotional distress or impaired functioning
   d. demonstration of a biological cause

3. Specific diagnostic criteria in DSM-III-R
   a. include essential features and associated features
   b. group behaviors according to their underlying causes
   c. are largely grouped according to psychodynamic theory
   d. are explanatory rather than descriptive

4. Maladaptive perceptions of others and their behaviors that have existed since childhood would be shown on axis _____ of DSM-III-R.
   a. I
   b. II
   c. IV
   d. V

5. Which of the following is a major <u>advantage</u> of DSM-III-R?
   a. eliminates multiple diagnosis
   b. high validity
   c. low reliability
   d. develops comprehensive view as a result of its multiaxial system

6. Which of the following is <u>not</u> a main approach to determining reliability?
   a. temporal stability
   b. interrater reliability
   c. internal consistency
   d. coefficient alpha

7. Criterion validity has two general types:
   a. content and concurrent
   b. construct and content
   c. concurrent and predictive
   d. construct and predictive

8. An interview which obtains identifying data, the client's description of the presenting problem, psychosocial and medical histories, current medical complaints and information about current medication is called
   a. a mental status examination
   b. a structured interview
   c. an unstructured interview
   d. a closed-ended interview

9. Which of the following is usually one of the judgments an interviewer makes in the mental status exam?
   a. reflection on emotional responses
   b. client's insight
   c. nature of the presenting problem
   d. level of client's rapport

10. Analogy: Paraphrasing is to reflection as
    a. thoughts are to emotions
    b. emotions are to thoughts
    c. summarization is to clarification
    d. intake interview is to mental status examination

11. The major value of the standardized interview is in
    a. its ability to produce high reliability without special training of interviewers
    b. minimizing interview time
    c. validity of diagnostic classification
    d. reliability of diagnostic classification

12. Abnormal behavior patterns are revealed on psychological tests by
    a. examination of validity scales to determine abnormal patterns of responding
    b. searching for extremely high scores
    c. comparing the client's responses to those made by groups of normal and abnormal individuals
    d. searching for extremely low scores

13. The Stanford-Binet Intelligence scale
    a. has recently been revised to produce an intelligence quotient
    b. was standardized for American children by Louis Terman
    c. is actually a series of separate tests for children and adults
    d. uses standard scores with a mean of 50 and standard deviation of 10

14. Which of the following is not true of research comparing IQs of people of various races and social classes?
    a. racial differences disappear when social class is held constant
    b. Black children typically score 15 to 20 points lower than White children
    c. many studies of IQ confound race with social class
    d. questions remain as to whether IQ differences reflect genetic differences among races or differences in cultural values

15. A personality assessment device in which the client is asked to make up a story about a house, tree and person is probably what type of test?
    a. neuropsychological
    b. intelligence
    c. self-report
    d. projective

16. Questions in the MMPI
    a. are open ended
    b. were selected because they discriminated between normal and clinical diagnostic populations
    c. were selected to detect individuals trying to "fake good"
    d. were chosen because they have a single correct answer

17. Performance of the _____ test of the Halstead-Reitan Neuropsychological Battery is believed to reflect functioning in the frontal lobe of the brain.
    a. category
    b. rhythm
    c. motor skills
    d. tactile performance

18. An assessment method which has the advantage of not relying on clients' self-reports but which may be distorted by attempts by the client to make a positive impression.
    a. self-monitoring using a wrist counter
    b. direct observation
    c. the behavioral rating scale
    d. measurement of the electrodermal response

19. A clinician who asks a series of questions about problem behaviors, their histories and their relationship to situational events is using which method of assessment?
    a. the mental status examination
    b. self-monitoring
    c. a behavioral checklist
    d. the behavioral interview

20. A client is recording the situation surrounding emotional states, and the category of disordered thinking that accompanied the emotional state. This client is using
    a. self-monitoring
    b. contrived measures
    c. a thought diary
    d. direct observation

21. Laing suggested that fear or anxiety consists of three different response systems:
    a. cognitive, emotional and physiological
    b. conscious, unconscious and preconscious
    c. behavioral, physiological and verbal
    d. behavioral, cognitive and subconscious

22. The two techniques for imaging the <u>activity</u> of various parts of the brain are
    a. NMR and BEAM
    b. PET and BEAM
    c. CAT and NMR
    d. EEG and NMR

TERMS AND CONCEPTS

Lesson 1
breadth of coverage (84)
clinical syndromes (81)
developmental disorders
(81)
DSM-III-R features (81)
global assessment of
functioning (82)
multiaxial (81)
personality disorders (81)
physical conditions and
disorders (82)
reliability of DSM-III (83)
severity of psychosocial
stressors (82)
validity of DSM-III (83)

Lesson 2
coefficient alpha (86)
concurrent validity (87)
construct validity (87)
content validity (86)
criterion validity (87)
internal consistency (86)
interrater reliability (86)
predictive validity (87)
reliability (86)
temporal stability (86)
validity (86)

Lesson 3
affect (90)
appearance (89)
behavioral observations
(89)
clarification (91)
insight (90)
intake interview (88)
intelligence (90)
memory (90)
mental status examination
(89)
orientation (90)
paraphrasing (91)
perceptual processes (90)
presenting problem (88)
rapport (89)
reflection (91)
sensorium (90)
structured interview (88)
summarization (91)
thought process (90)

Lesson 4
contrasted groups
approach (98)
deviation IQ (96)
Hermann Rorschach (102)
intelligence (95)

IQ (95)
Louis Terman (95)
MMPI (98)
neuropsychological
assessment (104)
Personality Tests (97)
projective tests (102)
psychological tests (93)
self-report (97)
self-report symptom
questionnaires (101)
standard scores (100)
Stanford-Binet Intelligence
Scale (95)
Thematic Apperception
Test (104)
validity scales (98)
Wechsler Scales (96)

Lesson 5
analogue measures (108)
BEAM (113)
behavioral assessment
(106)
behavioral interview (107)
behavioral rating scale
(110)
CAT scan (112)
cognitive assessment (110)
direct observation (109)
electrodermal response
(111)
electroencephalogram
(112)
electromyograph (114)
functional analysis (106)
NMR (113)
PET scan (112)
reactivity (108)
self-monitoring (107)

TYING THINGS TOGETHER

1. Do you (or should you) believe in astrology? Astrology attempts to predict personality characteristics and future life events based on your astrological sign. Psychologists claim that this is at best pseudoscience. What do you think? How might you decide? Here is your challenge: Clip the horoscope from your local paper. Make a list of the astrological advise (predictions) in random order without indicating which advise goes with which astrological

sign. Ask at least five friends to rate the accuracy of all of the predictions on the rating scale below. Then ask their birthdate to determine their sign. Does their seem to be a relationship between their sign and how accurate they said the information was? Are their more "false-positives" (accurate information but wrong sign) or more "true-negatives" (inaccurate information and wrong sign). Can you determine why people tend to believe in horoscope predictions?

<u>Rating Scale</u>
1. Definitely false   2. Mostly false   3. Mostly true   4. Definitely true

2.   Find out more about psychological tests. Visit your campus counseling center. Ask what kinds of tests they use when students come for help. How do they use the information to assist their clients? Perhaps your instructor would be willing to bring some samples of tests to class. Ask!

3.   Do you believe that self-monitoring is a reactive measure? Get a small notebook that you can carry in your pocket or purse and record some aspect of your behavior that you would like to change. Perhaps you would like to study more, lose weight (eat less), smoke less, swear less? You choose. The trick is to select a behavior that is easy to easily define and count. Record each behavior immediately after you do it. Keep a graph of your behavior versus days. A sample is provided below. Change "amount of behavior" to a more meaningful label ("Calories Eaten", "Hours of Study", "Cigarettes Smoked") Does your behavior change? Do you think that the act of self-monitoring is responsible? If you like the change, keep doing the self-monitoring. WMB was able to more than double his study time in graduate school by simply self-monitoring minutes studied.

Amount of Behavior

DAYS

Answers

Lesson 1
1 a
2 j
3 e
4 c
5 f
6 b
7 d
8 i
9 g
10 h
11 k

Lesson 2
1 c
2 j
3 h
4 k
5 g
6 a
7 f
8 e
9 b
10 d
11 i

Lesson 3
1 c
2 b
3 e
4 j
5 o
6 h
7 s
8 a
9 n
10 q
11 i
12 r
13 f
14 d
15 l
16 k
17 m
18 p
19 g

Lesson 4
1 d
2 f
3 i
4 c
5 j
6 o
7 g
8 r
9 b
10 k
11 m
12 h
13 a
14 p
15 e
16 n
17 l
18 q

Lesson 5
1 e
2 h
3 o
4 n
5 g
6 p
7 c
8 f
9 j
10 a
11 d
12 i
13 m
14 k
15 b
16 l

True-false answers
1 T
2 T
3 F
4 F
5 T
6 F
7 T
8 F
9 T
10 T
11 F
12 F
13 T
14 T
15 F
16 F
17 T
18 F
19 T
20 F
21 F
22 F

Multiple-Choice answers
1 b
2 c
3 a
4 b
5 d
6 d
7 c
8 b
9 b
10 a
11 d
12 c
13 b
14 a
15 d
16 b
17 a
18 b
19 d
20 c
21 c
22 b

4 Stress-Related Disorders

OVERVIEW

The chapter, "Stress Related Disorders," begins with the normal and ends with the abnormal. In this chapter, you will see that determining where normal ends and abnormal begins can be difficult. In spite of the difficulty in drawing the line between the two, you should be able to distinguish the end points. That is, you should know what constitutes normal, everyday sources of stress from abnormal, extraordinary sources of stress. You should also be able to distinguish normal and ordinary responses to stress from abnormal reactions to stress.

The chapter starts with a brief discussion of what stress is and points out that stress is not necessarily bad. A discussion of the major sources of stress follows. Events which produce stress include: the events and hassles of daily living; changes in our life circumstances; pain and physical discomfort; frustration from being unable to obtain goals; conflict over choosing between opposing goals; and the global environment. Stress from the global environment can be the result of on-going conditions, such as overcrowding, or from unique disasters, such as earthquakes, which threaten the control we have over our own lives.

After identifying what events produce stress, the chapter looks at the reactions produced by those stressful events. Stress produces both identifiable physiological and psychological reactions which are often related. These reactions to stress are greatly moderated by our expectations and responses as well as the responses of those around us.

The chapter ends with a consideration of the identification and treatment of two disorders defined in DSM-III-R, adjustment disorders and post-traumatic stress disorder. These are the first mental disorders covered in your text. Whenever you encounter a DSM-III-R disorder, your first task is to learn the diagnostic criteria for that disorder. The diagnostic criteria provide a functional definition of the disorder. DSM-III-R does not provide a separate category for stress-related disorders; however, stress is often a component of other disorders. Adjustment disorders are a class of maladaptive reactions, to specific stressful events, which impair work activity or social relationships. Post-traumatic stress disorder is impaired functioning following exposure to a disaster. The chapter ends with a brief discussion of treatments for stress-related disorders. These treatments focus on developing greater control of our responses.

CHAPTER OUTLINE, LESSONS & LEARNING OBJECTIVES

Lesson 1. Defining and identifying stress. (120-129)
STRESS. (120)
1. Define stress.
SOURCES OF STRESS. (120-129)
2. Identify the sources of stress.
3. Describe research about the relationship between daily hassles, life events, and illness.

Lesson 2. Responding to stress. (129-131)
RESPONSES TO STRESS. (129-131)
4. Describe the three stages of the general adaptation syndrome (GAS).
5. Explain how the endocrine system and the autonomic nervous system react in each stage of the GAS.
6. Describe emotional responses to stress.
7. Describe psychological methods for lowering arousal.

Lesson 3. Factors altering the response to stress. (131-140)
PSYCHOLOGICAL MODERATORS OF THE IMPACT OF STRESS. (131-140)
8. Explain how self-efficacy expectancies, psychological hardiness, humor, whether one is a goal-directed or playful mode, predictability, and social support moderate the effects of stress.
9. Explain how social support, life expectancy, and the stress of natural and technological disasters interrelate.

Lesson 4. Abnormal reactions to stress and their treatment. (140-147)
ADJUSTMENT DISORDERS. (140-141)
10. Identify the essential features of adjustment disorders.
11. Explain why labeling an adjustment disorder as a "mental disorder" blurs the line between what is normal and what is abnormal.
POST-TRAUMATIC STRESS DISORDER. (141-145)
12. Identify the essential features of PTSD.
13. Explain why Vietnam war veterans are more likely to suffer from PTSD than veterans of other wars.
14. Describe the conditioning theory of PTSD and approaches to treatment.
TREATMENT OF STRESS-RELATED DISORDERS. (145-147)
15. Describe treatments for stress-related disorders.

Mastering Lesson 1. Defining and identifying stress. (120-129)

This lesson is relatively straightforward. It has a simple goal, to provide you with the information necessary to give a coherent and complete response to the question, "what is stress?" Although you may have a clear idea of what you mean by "stress", you need to know what psychologists mean when they refer to "stress" or "stressors".

First, you will memorize definitions for two basic terms, stress and eustress. These terms define the basic topic of the chapter. Then, you will need to learn what produces stress and eustress. The chapter discusses five basic and complimentary approaches to identifying stressors. (Stressors are events which produce stress.) The first is Lazarus' examination of unavoidable and unpleasant daily events which produce stress. The second is Holmes & Rahe's examination of life changes, both bad and good, which produce stress. The third is an analysis of pain. The fourth is an analysis of frustration and conflict; the fifth, a brief analysis of disasters.

You should learn a basic description of Lazarus' and Holmes & Rahe's approaches as well as some concrete examples of the events that these approaches cover. You should also be able to summarize the research on the correlation between the amount of life change individuals experience correlates and physical illness. You will need to know the physiological reactions produced by painful stimuli and the six basic techniques used to reduce reactivity to painful stimuli. You should be able to define the terms frustration and conflict and describe the four basic types of conflict. Finally, you will need to be able to distinguish between natural and technological disasters.

Match the following terms and concepts with the correct definitions or description or explanation.

1. __ 150 or less LCUs
2. __ 300 or more LCUs
3. __ analgesics
4. __ approach-approach conflict
5. __ approach-avoidance conflict
6. __ avoidance-avoidance conflict
7. __ conflict
8. __ daily hassles
9. __ endorphins
10. __ environmental hassles
11. __ eustress
12. __ events with high life change units
13. __ events with low life change units
14. __ financial responsibility hassles
15. __ frustration
16. __ future security hassles
17. __ health hassles
18. __ Holmes & Rahe
19. __ household hassles
20. __ inner-concern hassles
21. __ life-change unit
22. __ multiple approach-avoidance conflict
23. __ natural disaster
24. __ prostaglandin
25. __ six basic techniques of pain reduction
26. __ stress
27. __ survivor guilt
28. __ technological disaster
29. __ time-pressure hassles
30. __ work hassles

a. 30% chance of developing medical problems
b. 80% chance of developing medical problems
c. a neurotransmitter which blocks pain messages in the nervous system
d. a measure of the importance of various changes in one's life
e. air pollution, traffic congestion, noise and crime
f. an event requiring one to adjust, cope, or adapt
g. chemical released at the site of a physical injury
h. choosing among goals all of which have positive and negative aspects
i. Christmas and vacation
j. concerns about job security and retirement
k. concerns about debts or sending children to college
l. divorce, marriage, death of a family member
m. everyday incidents that threaten a person's well-being
n. feelings of loneliness and concern about the meaning of life
o. frustration which results when opposing motives are a barrier
p. having too much to do and not enough time
q. inhibit production of prostaglandin
r. life changes as sources of stress
s. making meals, shopping, and house cleaning
t. problems with supervisors and co-workers
u. providing accurate information, distraction & fantasy, hypnosis, relaxation training, coping with irrational beliefs, and social support
v. sickness and concern about health
w. stress leading to desirable changes
x. the result of thwarting or blocking goals or needs
z. disaster for which one can be blamed
aa. disaster for which no can be blamed
bb. a single goal with positive and negative outcomes
cc. trying to attain two different positive goals
dd. choosing between two different negative goals
ee. negative feelings experienced by those who survive disasters

Mastering Lesson 2. Responding to stress. (129-131)

This section looks at three ways in which we can respond to the stressors discussed in Lesson 1. The primary focus is on physiological reactions and, more specifically, the general adaptation syndrome (GAS). An understanding of the GAS will require you to know the names and the sequence of the three stages of the GAS. You will also need to be able to know the relationship among the three GAS stages, the sympathetic nervous system, and the endocrine system. Although most of these bodily changes are not easily perceived, you should try to remember or notice how your body responds to stress. This will help make this abstract material more meaningful to you.

Those reactions to stress which are more easily recognized are the three emotional reactions which are discussed next. You will quickly recognize these emotions in your own reactions to stress. This section ends with an extended discussion of mediation and progressive relaxation as methods to reduce the effect of stressors, that is, make us experience less stress. After carefully reading about each technique, practice using each technique, at least, once. This will not only insure that you will remember everything you need to know about each technique but you will also learn something that can be valuable in your own life. For example, engaging in progressive relaxation before an exam can reduce anxiety which interferes with exam performance.

Match the following terms and concepts with the correct definition or description or explanation.

1. __ alarm reaction
2. __ anger
3. __ anxiety
4. __ depression
5. __ exhaustion stage
6. __ GAS
7. __ GAS stage with cardiovascular and muscle fatigue
8. __ GAS stage with high epinephrine & sugar levels
9. __ GAS stage with moderate endocrine and sympathetic levels
10. __ Hans Selye
11. __ mantra
12. __ meditation
13. __ progressive relaxation
14. __ resistance stage
15. __ Walter Cannon

a. a relaxing sound used in transcendental meditation
b. alarm reaction
c. an emotion consisting of a generalized sense of fear or apprehension
d. an emotion of mixed sympathetic and parasympathetic activity
e. an emotion similar to the exhaustion stage of the GAS
f. coined the expression fight-or-flight syndrome
g. coined the expression general adaptation syndrome
h. exhaustion stage
i. general adaptation syndrome
j. method to increase awareness and control of muscular tension and relaxation
k. mobilizes the body for action through activation of sympathetic system
l. narrowing consciousness to moderate our sense of the outer world
m. period when body attempts to restore energy and repair damage
n. resistance stage
o. the parasympathetic system dominates the sympathetic system

Mastering Lesson 3. Factors altering the response to stress. (131-140)

So far, this chapter has dealt with the way in which reactions to stressors are constant. This lesson focuses on two factors which alter the response to stress: an individual's personality and the social environment in which the stress occurs.

Your text discusses four major personality dimensions which affect our reactions to stressors. Self-efficacy expectancies are the degree to which a person believes she or he can cope with problems and adopt new behaviors to solve problems. Persons with high self-efficacy are less disturbed by stress. Psychological hardiness is a combination of three individual differences or personality characteristics which contribute to better stress management. The most important of these is locus of control, which is the degree to which we believe we control our own lives. An "internal" person believes they control their life and is less trouble by stress. An "external' person believes that chance controls their life.

The concepts of self-efficacy and locus of control are related but different. You should pay attention to the differences between these two concepts and, in particular, the difference in the way in which the two characteristics are measured. [You may find that you have trouble distinguishing the two concepts. If you do, ask your instructor for help. This is a difficult distinction for psychologists to understand, so you won't be alone.]

The last two personality dimensions your text considers is humor and goal-directedness versus playfulness. Although these characteristics may be stable in some persons, in other persons, they are highly situational. That is, some people are constantly goal-directed or playful, while other people may be serious or playful depending upon the situation. These two topics provide a transition to two important situational variables which alter the influence of stressors.

Predictability refers to an individual's ability to predict and control the occurrence of stressors. Social support refers to the reactions to us when we experience stress.

Match the following terms and concepts with the correct definitions or description or explanation.

1. __ goal directed
2. __ high self-efficacy
3. __ humor
4. __ locus of control
5. __ playful
6. __ predictability
7. __ psychological hardiness
8. __ self-efficacy expectancies
9. __ social support
10. __ Weiss

a. a person's belief that they control their lives
b. a person's beliefs about their ability to cope or to change
c. a state in which onset and intensity of stressors is known
d. a state of seriousness in which high arousal is stressful
e. a state of spontaneous activity in which high arousal is not stressful
f. associated with lower levels of epinephrine in the bloodstream
g. emotional concern, instrumental aid, information, appraisal & socializing
h. high levels of commitment, challenge, and perceived control
i. rats who could not control and predict shocks developed ulcers.
j. using a jest to provide a buffer to the effects of stress

Mastering Lesson 4. Abnormal reactions to stress. (140-147)

This lessons covers the first two disorders from DSM-III-R. The diagnostic criteria of these two disorders are relatively simple. So use this lesson to practice for the more difficult disorders to follow in later chapters.

The best way to learn diagnostic criteria is to make a list of the criteria for each disorder. You will need to pay particular attention to those criteria that distinguish one disorder from another. Once you are sure what the criteria are, look over the examples presented in you text and identify the important diagnostic criteria in the example. If you are unsure about your diagnosis, consult your instructor.

Match the following terms and concepts with the correct definitions or description or explanation.

1. __ adjustment disorder
2. __ battle fatigue
3. __ behavior therapy
4. __ conditioning model of PTSD
5. __ post traumatic stress disorder
6. __ stress inoculation therapy

a. a temporary, maladaptive reaction to an identified stressor
b. old term for PTSD due to exposure to combat
c. reexperiencing a extraordinary, distressing event
d. reexposure to cues associated with a trauma without the trauma
e. training to relax in anticipation of encountering stressors
f. traumatic experiences become associated with neutral reccurring stimuli

PRACTICE EXAM

Exam 1. (true-false)

Indicate whether each of the following statements is **True** or **False**. Question numbers correspond to learning objectives from which the questions were drawn.

1. __ Stress is the negative impact caused by life events.
2. __ Life changes are more isolated events than daily hassles.
3. __ Evidence clearly shows that life changes cause physical illness.
4. __ Resistance is the second stage of the GAS.
5. __ Sugar is released by the liver during the exhaustion stage of the GAS.
6. __ High levels of arousal facilitate finding adaptive responses.
7. __ Mediation decreases arousal by focusing on a single stimulus.
8. __ External locus of control leads to psychological hardiness.
9. __ Women who watch less television live longer.
10. __ With an adjustment disorder, the maladaptive behavior occurs for longer than six months.
11. __ With an adjustment disorder, a clinician must determine if a behavior exceeds an expectable level.
12. __ Persons suffering from PTSD are more responsive to normal events than other people.
13. __ Vietnam veterans have a higher incidence of PTSD than other veterans of the same age.
14. __ PTSD can be easily treated with tranquilizers such as valium.

49

15.__ A behavior therapist would expose a victim of PTSD to traumatic stimuli as a therapy.

Exam 2 (multiple-choice)

Select the single, best answer for each question. Question numbers correspond to learning objectives from which the questions were drawn.

1. Hans Selye coined the term _____ to refer to small or moderate amounts of stress which helps maintain alertness.
   a. malstress
   b. ameliostress
   c. activating stress
   d. eustress

2. Lazarus calls the stress induced by the responsibility of cooking meals, family shopping, and house keeping
   a. household hassles
   b. housewife stress syndrome
   c. time-pressure hassles
   d. environmental hassle

3. Which of the following events is less than 50 life-change units (LCUs) on the Holmes and Rahe scale?
   a. marriage
   b. divorce
   c. personal illness
   d. pregnancy

4. The correct order of stages in the general adaptation syndrome (GAS) is
   a. exhaustion, alarm, resistance
   b. alarm, exhaustion, resistance
   c. alarm, resistance, exhaustion
   d. resistance, alarm, exhaustion

5. Which of the following occurs during the alarm stage of the GAS?
   a. blood pressure drops
   b. muscle tension increases
   c. respiration rates decline
   d. epinephrine levels decrease

6. The emotional reaction to stress which is characterized by rapid heart rate, rapid breathing, sweating, and general muscular tension is
   a. anxiety
   b. anger
   c. depression
   d. repulsion

7. Using a **mantra** to reduce tension is a technique of
   a. progressive relaxation
   b. cognitive-behavior therapy
   c. stress-inoculation training
   d. transcendental meditation

8. Under which of the following circumstances were rats <u>most</u> likely to develop ulcers in Weiss's experiments on predictability and control of stressful events?
   a. rats given no signal and no shock
   b. rats given a signal but no control
   c. rats given a signal and control
   d. rats given no signal and no control

9. Telling a person whether or not she or he is handling a stressor well is providing which kind of social support for that person?
   a. appraisal
   b. emotional concern
   c. information
   d. socializing

10. All but one of the following is one of the diagnostic criteria for an adjustment disorder. Indicate which symptom is <u>not</u> one of the criteria for diagnosing an adjustment disorder.
    a. maladaptive reaction to an unidentifiable source
    b. impaired ability to do ones job
    c. inability to engage in normal social activity
    d. reactions in excess of what would be expected

11. Which of the following statements is true about diagnosing adjustment disorders?
    a. Diagnosing adjustment disorders is easy because clinicians believe that people should face disasters with a "happy face".
    b. Adjustment disorders consist of behavioral disturbance without any emotional disturbance.
    c. The most common adjustment disorder is the Adjustment Disorder with Biphasic Mood Swings.
    d. With a severe stressor, a normal reaction may be so maladaptive that it is diagnosed as an adjustment disorder.

12. Which of the following symptoms is <u>not</u> one of the diagnostic criteria for PTSD?
    a. decreased appetite and weight loss
    b. strong feelings of detachment
    c. recurrent nightmares about the traumatic event
    d. irritability or angry outbursts

13. The higher incidence of PTSD among Vietnam veterans may occur because Vietnam veterans
    a. are older than veterans of other wars
    b. were more likely to experience combat than other veterans
    c. were not welcomed home to large public celebrations
    d. faced a more readily identifiable enemy

14. According to the classical conditioning model of PTSD, traumatic experiences act as a(n)
   a. conditioned response
   b. unconditioned response
   c. conditioned stimulus
   d. unconditioned stimulus
15. Putting clients in stressful situations to try out stress reducing behaviors is a technique of
   a. psychoanalysis
   b. person-centered therapy
   c. cognitive-behavior therapy
   d. self therapy

TERMS AND CONCEPTS

Lesson 1
150 or less LCUs (121)
300 or more LCUs (121)
analgesics (125)
approach-approach conflict (127)
approach-avoidance conflict (127)
avoidance-avoidance conflict (127)
conflict (126)
daily hassles (120)
endorphins (125)
environmental hassles (120)
eustress (120)
events with high life change units (121)
events with low life change units (121)
financial responsibility hassles (120)
frustration (126)
future security hassles (120)
health hassles (120)
Holmes & Rahe (121)
household hassles (120)
inner-concern hassles (120)
life-change unit (121)
multiple approach-avoidance conflict (127)
natural disaster (128)
prostaglandin (125)
six basic techniques of pain reduction (125)
stress (120)
survivor guilt (128)
technological disaster (128)
time-pressure hassles (120)
work hassles (120)

Lesson 2
alarm reaction (129)
anger (131)
anxiety (131)
depression (131)
exhaustion stage (130)
GAS (129)
GAS stage with cardiovascular and muscle fatigue (130)
GAS stage with high epinephrine & sugar levels (129)
GAS stage with moderate endocrine and sympathetic levels (130)
Hans Selye (129)
mantra (132)
meditation (132)
progressive relaxation (133)
resistance stage (130)
Walter Cannon (129)

Lesson 3
goal directed (135)
high self-efficacy (131)
humor (134)
locus of control (134)
playful (135)
predictability (135)
psychological hardiness (134)
self-efficacy expectancies (131)
social support (138)
Weiss (135)

Lesson 4
adjustment disorder (140)
battle fatigue (143)
behavior therapy (145)
conditioning model of PTSD (145)
post traumatic stress disorder (141)
stress inoculation therapy (145)

TYING THINGS TOGETHER

1. It is quite likely you or someone you have encountered someone has suffered from an adjustment disorder. Using a pseudonym, write a brief psychological report for this person. Your report should include a brief biographical sketch; a description of the precipitating event(s); a description of the specific behaviors indicative of an adjustment disorder; and a specific diagnosis (see Table 4.3 in your text).

2. Rape victims are often subject to the development of Post-Traumatic Stress Disorder. What changes in society could be made to reduce PTSD in rape victims and why would they work?

3. The most personally valuable piece of information you will find in your text is the set of instructions on how to do progressive relaxation. Using you own voice, record the progressive relaxation instructions on a cassette tape recorder. Read the instructions slowly and in an even tone of voice. Once you have made the recording listen to and follow the instructions at the same time every day for five days. Record, as if in a diary, how you feel each day after you have practiced relaxing.

ANSWERS

Lesson 1	Lesson 2	Lesson 3	Lesson 4
1 a	1 k	1 d	1 a
2 b	2 d	2 f	2 b
3 q	3 c	3 j	3 c
4 cc	4 e	4 a	4 f
5 bb	5 o	5 e	5 c
6 dd	6 i	6 c	6 e
7 o	7 h	7 h	
8 m	8 b	8 b	
9 c	9 n	9 g	
10 e	10 g	10 i	
11 w	11 a		
12 l	12 l		
13 i	13 j		
14 k	14 m		
15 x	15 f		
16 j			
17 v			
18 r			
19 s			
20 n			
21 d			
22 h			
23 aa			
24 g			
25 u			
26 f			
27 ee			
28 z			
29 p			
30 t			

True-False answers

1 F	11 T
2 T	12 T
3 F	13 T
4 T	14 F
5 F	15 T
6 F	
7 T	
8 F	
9 T	
10 F	

Multiple-Choice answers

1 b	11 d
2 a	12 a
3 c	13 c
4 c	14 d
5 b	15 c
6 a	
7 d	
8 d	
9 a	
10 a	

5 Psychological Factors and Health

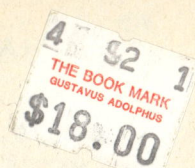

OVERVIEW

If you have gotten comfortable thinking in terms of the medical model of abnormal behavior, this chapter may turn your viewpoint upside down. While the medical model focused on internal, often physical, causes of abnormal behavior, this chapter focuses on behavioral causes of (and sometimes treatment for) physical health problems. Psychological factors are related to health in a variety of ways that you will encounter in this chapter. Psychological factors can play a direct, causal role in health problems, they can play an indirect role when behavior results in unnecessary exposure to risk factors for major health problems, or the behavior itself may be a risk factor.

The chapter begins with a bit of a flair for the exciting. After summarizing the rather dramatic self-reported case study of Norman Cousins, the text focuses on immune system function can be altered by psychological factors, not something we usually consider. After discussing psychological factors involved in headaches and their treatment and menstrual problems, the chapter moves to the circulatory system and two of the most serious public health problems today, hypertension and coronary heart disease. Following discussions of psychological factors in ulcers, asthma and cancer the chapter turns to AIDS as an epidemic whose spread is largely controllable by altering sexually motivated behavior--a problem with which clinicians from the learning perspective are well-equipped to deal. The final section deals with obesity, itself a risk factor for coronary heart disease, from the perspective of psychological factors implicated in its development and the effectiveness of including psychological principles in weight loss programs.

In the larger perspective of the chapter you should recognize the wide range of health problems that are affected, either directly or indirectly, by psychological factors. You might even begin to wonder if there are any health problems where psychological factors are _not_ important. Clearly there are a lot of topics in this chapter. Much to be learned, but so few pages to tell you about all of it. Thus, you should expect that the important ideas in this chapter are packed in tightly. Pay attention to detail as you read. You should find more important things per page than you did in the early chapters.

CHAPTER OUTLINE, LESSONS & LEARNING OBJECTIVES

Lesson 1.   Psychological factors in physical health, the immune system. (150-156)
PSYCHOLOGICAL FACTORS AFFECTING PHYSICAL CONDITION. (150-153)
1.   Explain ways in which psychological factors affect our physical condition.
THE IMMUNE SYSTEM. (153-156)
2.   Explain the functions of the immune system.
3.   Explain the effects of stress on the immune system.

Lesson 2.   Common pain: Headaches and menstrual problems. (156-160)
HEADACHES. (156-157)
4.   Differentiate between tension headaches and migraine headaches.
5.   Summarize research attempting to identify origins of various types of headaches.
6.   Describe biological and psychological treatments for headache.
MENSTRUAL PROBLEMS. (157-160)
7.   Describe various kinds of menstrual problems.
8.   Describe theory and research concerned with the origins of menstrual problems.

Lesson 3.   The circulatory system: Hypertension and cardiovascular disorders. (160-169)
HYPERTENSION. (160-161)
9.   Describe the theory and research concerning the origins of essential hypertension.
10.   Describe biological and psychological approaches to managing hypertension
CARDIOVASCULAR DISORDERS. (161-169)
11.   List and briefly describe the major risk factors for coronary heart disease.
12.   Understand the Type A behavior pattern and research relating it to coronary heart disease.
13.   Describe ways in which modifying behavior can reduce coronary heart disease risk.

Lesson 4.   Gastrointestinal disorders, asthma cancer and AIDS. (169-178)
GASTROINTESTINAL DISORDERS. (169-172)
14.   Discuss the theoretical perspective on ulcers.
ASTHMA. (172-173)
15.   Discuss the theoretical perspectives on asthma.
CANCER. (173-175)
16.   List and briefly describe the risk factors for cancer.
17.   Discuss research findings investigating psychological factors in the course and treatment of cancer.
ACQUIRED IMMUNE DEFICIENCY SYNDROME (AIDS). (175-178)
18.   Discuss the biological and psychological effects of AIDS.
19.   Discuss roles for psychologists in the prevention and treatment of AIDS.

Lesson 5.   Obesity and its treatment. (178-186)
OBESITY. (178-186)
20.   Discuss theoretical perspectives on obesity.
21.   Summarize research concerning treatments of obesity.

Mastering Lesson 1. Psychological factors in physical health, the immune system. (150-156)

This lesson introduces the relationships between psychological factors and health; then the first of these relationships, that of the immune system and stress is described. We usually think of the immune system as having basically an automatic function that is totally under biological control. Recent research in psychoneuroimmunology, which most of us don't hear about, has clearly laid that oversimplification to rest. In learning the material pay attention to how it is organized, for most of the remainder of the chapter will be organized similarly. Rathus and Nevid first introduce a topic, in this case that includes giving you some needed background about the biology of the immune system. Then they tell you about the empirical research on that topic. They usually (but not this time) explain contemporary theoretical views of the underlying causal relationships, and end with a brief discussion of research on treatment issues. Expecting this organization should make your learning more efficient and the matching section below should help you learn the essential terminology of the lesson.

Match the following terms and concepts with the correct definition or description or explanation.

1. E antibodies
2. A antigens
3. D diathesis-stress model
4. G immune system
5. B inflammation
6. C leukocytes
7. F psychoneuro-
      immunology

a. antibody generators
b. caused by increased blood flow to injured area
c. white blood cells, they search and destroy pathogens
d. stress combines with genetic predisposition (diathesis) to produce a behavior disorder
e. proteins produced by leukocytes that identify and destroy antigens
f. interdisciplinary field concerned with psychological factors and the immune system
g. system for recognizing and destroying pathogens that enter our bodies

Mastering Lesson 2. Common pain: Headaches and menstrual problems. (156-160)

Headaches are categorized as (muscle) tension and other (including migraine). You will learn to distinguish headache type by its cause, describe the causes of headache including psychological factors, summarize basic treatment methods and describe the results of some treatment outcome studies.

The second topic in this lesson is menstrual problems. In this component you will learn about pain associated with menstrual cycles, and how that pain can be treated. Premenstrual syndrome (PMS) also called late luteal phase disorder, is also included in this lesson. Notice the conflicting research and theoretical perspectives on PMS. We should note that both men and women have much to gain personally from this part of the lesson. Although many women do not directly experience the problems in this section and men may feel that they are irrelevant, all of us have known or will know someone who is affected. Understanding the biological and psychological factors involved in menstrual problems can help all of us to be more understanding of these individuals. The matching section that follows will begin to develop this understanding.

Match the following terms and concepts with the correct definition or description or explanation.

B 1. **B** dysmenorrhea
D 2. **D** electromyographic biofeedback
  3. **A** estradiol and progesterone
  4. **G** ibuprofen
  5. **F** individual response specificity
  6. **I** migraine headache
  7. **J** premenstrual syndrome
H 8. **H** prostaglandins
  9. **E** tension headache
C 10. **C** thermal biofeedback

a. hormones implicated in PMS
b. general menstrual pain or discomfort
c. a biofeedback technique for migraine headaches
d. a biofeedback technique for preventing tension headaches
e. gradually developing, dull steady pain resulting from stress-induced muscle contraction
f. stressors have different effects due to genetic factors, learning history and encoding
g. inhibits production of prostaglandins involved in transmission of pain messages
h. copious secretions during and prior to menstruation may explain pain and discomfort
i. intense, piercing pain resulting from changes in blood flow to the brain
j. characterized by irritability, weight gain, depression and abdominal discomfort usually confined to the four days prior to menstruation

T—MI
MY—TEN

Mastering Lesson 3. The circulatory system: Hypertension and (HIGH BLOOD PRESSURE) cardiovascular disorders. (160-169)

In this lesson you will learn about psychological factors in two serious public health problems: hypertension and cardiovascular disorders. Notice that suspected psychological factors in hypertension are related to the psychodynamic and learning theoretical perspectives.

Since cardiovascular disorders are our number one source of death, much research has been devoted to understanding, treating and preventing cardiovascular disorders. A number of risk factors for coronary heart disease (CHD) have emerged from this research. These are variables that place the individual at higher risk for CHD. Except for *age*, *sex* and *family history*, these risk factors are all lifestyle factors. That is, we can change them by altering aspects of our lifestyle. In this lesson you will learn the risk factors for CHD and how changing the lifestyle factors can reduce CHD risk. One of these risk factors, *Type A Behavior Pattern* (TABP), is a personality characteristic that is singled out for greater depth of coverage. You will learn about it, some of the debate surrounding research linking TABP to CHD, and treatments to attempt to alter Type A Behavior. Emotion-focused coping and problem-focused coping are two major ways in which people deal with environmental stressors. These are also given more attention in the chapter. The matching section provides you with an opportunity to learn the technical vocabulary that is new to this section.

Match the following terms and concepts with the correct definition or description or explanation.

1. **D** aerobic exercise
2. **A** anaerobic exercise
3. **F** arteriosclerosis
4. **H** atherosclerosis
5. **E** cardiovascular disorders
6. **J** CHD risk factors
7. **G** coronary heart disease
8. **L** dietary treatment of hypertension
9. **I** emotion-focused coping
10. **K** essential hypertension
11. **B** problem-focused coping
12. **C** Type A Behavior

a. weight training
b. coping by altering environment to reduce stressors
c. impatient, competitive and aggressive describe it
d. running or cycling
e. coronary heart disease, hypertension and atherosclerosis
f. thickening and hardening of the arteries
g. leading cause of death for men over 40 and women over 70
h. deposition of fatty substances along walls of arteries
i. coping by pretending the problem does not exist
j. obesity, Type A Personality, smoking, inactivity are just a few
k. high blood pressure for which there is no identifiable physical cause
l. low sodium and weight loss are the two primary ones

Mastering Lesson 4. Gastrointestinal disorders, asthma, cancer and AIDS. (169-178)

This lesson combines four short sections from the textbook. In mastering the first two of these sections, you should focus on the role of stress as a causal factor or as a factor that exacerbates ulcers and asthma suffering when combined with other factors. The section on cancer differs. Here you should focus primarily on how stress can affect the course (progression) of cancer and how psychological treatments can be used to enhance the effectiveness of medical treatment. The psychologist's roles in AIDS includes helping individuals alter their lifestyles to prevent transmission of AIDS and providing psychological help to individuals who are already infected. Much of this lesson focuses on relationships and background research. There is less new terminology to master, hence the matching section is relatively short.

Match the following terms and concepts with the correct definition or description or explanation.

1. **A** AIDS
2. **H** AIDS risks
3. **C** asthma
4. **D** coping skills training
5. **G** immune surveillance theory
6. **E** pepsin
7. **B** peptic ulcers
8. **E** taste aversions

a. estimated to affect nearly 1.5 million Americans
b. two types are gastric and duodenal
c. allergic reaction which constricts bronchi
d. a psychological adjunct to cancer treatment that includes cognitive and behavioral methods
e. pairing specific food with gastric distress
f. breaks down proteins; responsible for peptic ulcers
g. failure of immune system to destroy mutant cells causes cancer
h. male homosexuality, intravenous drug use, blood transfusions, to mention only three

Mastering Lesson 5. Obesity and its treatment. (178-186)

Obesity is not only a problem in its own right, but is also a risk factor for CHD. Considerable research by a variety of disciplines has helped us to understand more about feeding and metabolism and how they lead to the development of obesity. Thus the theoretical perspectives component has a variety of viewpoints represented. Psychologists have devoted considerable research effort to development of effective treatment programs. Thus there are two major objectives in this lesson. The matching section below will help you become facile with the theories of obesity and methods of treating it.

Match the following terms and concepts with the correct definition or description or explanation.

1. M appetite suppressing drugs
2. H changing antecedents
3. C changing behaviors
4. O changing consequences
5. A eating as oral fixation
6. I external eaters
7. G fat cells
8. K internal eaters
9. F metabolic rate
10. D self-control behavioral treatment
11. L set point
12. G stop center
13. B surgical treatments for obesity
14. E VLCD
15. N yo-yo syndrome

a. psychodynamic viewpoint
b. intestinal bypass and liposuction are two examples
c. putting down utensils between bites
d. produces modest weight loss but good maintenance
e. lower metabolic rate resulting from repeated food restriction
f. a major means of hereditary transmission of obesity
g. destruction of this produces hyperphagia in rats
h. eat on a smaller plate
i. food stimuli are primary signals to eat
j. metabolize food more slowly than muscle
k. eat primarily in response to hunger
l. level of fat cell size depletion that triggers hunger drive
m. enhance weight loss but negatively associated with long term maintenance
n. consuming 300-600 calories daily produces rapid weight loss that is quickly regained
o. sending a dollar to the most despicable person you know when you eat chocolate cake

PRACTICE EXAMS

Exam 1. (true-false).
Indicate whether each of the following statements is True or False. Question numbers correspond to learning objectives from which the questions were drawn.

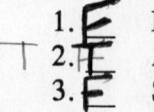

1. F Psychophysiological disorders are psychological problems due to biological tissue damage.
2. T F Antigens stimulate the production of antibodies which lead to destruction of the antigens.
3. F Stress results in increased steroid production which increases the activity of the immune system.
4. F F Tension headaches are often preceded by an aura such as flashing lights.
5. T Modern theory suggests that migraine headaches are caused by dysfunctional regulation of serotonin in the brain.

62

6. F Treatment of tension headaches using biofeedback involves providing patients with information about blood flow in peripheral limbs to allow them to learn to control their bodily distribution of blood flow.

7. T PMS symptoms generally preceded menstruation by up to four days.

8. T While estradiol and progesterone levels are thought to be implicated in PMS, research has been inconclusive

9. T According to psychodynamic theory, essential hypertension results from pent-up feelings of hostility and anger.

10. F Research by Blanchard showed that thermal biofeedback was less effective than relaxation training in the treatment of hypertension.

11. F Even low to moderate alcohol consumption increases the risk of CHD.

12. T Heart attack victims with Type A Behavior Pattern are less likely to die of a subsequent heart attack than are victims with Type B Behavior Pattern.

13. F Providing health information on diet, exercise and medical problems is effective in reducing CHD risk.

14. F According to the biological perspective, somatic expression of psychosexual conflict is a major cause of ulcers.

15. F Children who died from asthma were shown to be more likely to suffer from depression indicating a causal role for psychological factors.

16. T Most risk factors for cancer involve behavior patterns which can be changed.

17. F Calm, cool, collected emotional states offer the best prognosis for cancer survival.

18. T HIV depletes T4 lymphocytes allowing opportunistic diseases to develop.

19. T Education alone is insufficient to reduce AIDS risk behaviors; it must be supplemented with effective behavior change assistance.

20. F Women have a lower percentage of body fat than men and therefore require fewer calories of food to maintain their weight.

21. T Behavior modification treatments focus on the ABCs of eating.

Exam 2 (multiple-choice)

Select the single, best answer for each question. Question numbers correspond to learning objectives from which the questions were drawn.

1. DSM-III-R includes the relationship of physical health factors to psychological factors by
   a. listing the physical condition on Axis III
   b. including psychological factors affecting physical condition on Axis I
   c. both a and b
   d. neither a nor b

2. Leukocytes
   a. produce antigens to identify pathogens
   b. cause inflammation of injured areas
   c. are foreign invaders in our bodies such as bacteria, viruses and fungi
   d. form the basis of the body's immune response

3. The experiment by Weiss (1972) in which rats were shocked showed that suppression of the immune system occurred in
   a. all rats who were shocked
   b. rats who could not do anything to terminate shocks
   c. rats who could control the ending of the shocks
   d. control rats who observed other rats being shocked

4. Headaches characterized by dull, steady pain on both sides of the head are
   a. caused by serotonin disregulation
   b. called tension headaches
   c. caused by problems with blood flow to the brain
   d. often preceded by an aura

5. Some individuals develop tension headaches when subjected to stress while others do not. The reason for this is
   a. related to prostaglandin levels
   b. found in principle of individual response specificity
   c. found in serotonin dysfunction
   d. presently unknown

6. Aspirin and ibuprofen relieve pain by
   a. inhibiting production of prostaglandins
   b. increasing production of prostaglandins
   c. inhibition of serotonin production
   d. inhibition of estradiol production

7. Menstrual pain and late luteal phase disorder are
   a. both examples of dysmenorrhea
   b. caused by prostaglandin secretion
   c. caused by estradiol levels
   d. causes of depression

8. We now know that research by Dalton exaggerated the extent of menstrual problems. More recent research has shown that
   a. only about 30% of college women report menstrual symptoms that impair their academic performance
   b. suicides among adult females were three times less likely to occur during menstruation
   c. the diagnosis of PMS stigmatizes patients and should therefore be avoided
   d. fewer than 1% of employed women miss work because of menstrual problems

9. From a biological perspective, essential hypertension is viewed as
   a. the result of constricted blood vessels due to organic disease
   b. cardiovascular response to pent-up feelings of anger and hostility
   c. the result of the cardiovascular system overreacting to stress
   d. the result of dilated blood vessels due to organic disease

10. Low sodium and weight loss diets in the treatment of hypertension
    a. are effective by themselves for over 70% of patients
    b. must be supplemented by anti-hypertensive medication
    c. are less effective than biofeedback training
    d. must be combined with relaxation training or biofeedback to help a majority of patients

11. Which of the following is not true of smoking as a CHD risk factor?
    a. smokers have about double the risk of death from CHD as compared to nonsmokers
    b. CHD risk can be reduced up to 50 percent in people who quit smoking prior to age 65
    c. the longer an ex-smoker remains abstinent, the lower his/her CHD risk becomes
    d. CHD risk from smoking is independent of stress level

12. Although the final answer is not in, current research on Type A Behavior Pattern seems to suggest that CHD is
    a. related only to the aggressiveness component of TABP
    b. related only to the hostility component of TABP
    c. related only to the impatience component of TABP
    d. unrelated to TABP

13. CHD risk can be reduced by
    a. engaging in anaerobic exercise, but not by aerobic exercise
    b. the use of emotion-focused coping skills
    c. eating diets high in coconut and palm oils but not by anaerobic exercise
    d. seeking increased personal control over productivity in the workplace

14. The case of Tom, the individual with a plastic window in his stomach, provides support for
    a. the psychodynamic explanation of ulcers
    b. the biological perspective of ulcer development
    c. the stimulus specificity view of ulcer development
    d. the individual response specificity explanation of ulcer development

15. Asthma attacks can be induced by
    a. any stress of sufficient intensity
    b. fear of airflow restriction
    c. stress induced by physical injury
    d. any irrational fear of sufficient intensity

16. The best conclusion about the relation of stress to the development of cancer which can be drawn from current information is that
    a. stress may affect the timing of cancer onset but not its eventual outcome
    b. cancer is the cause of stress rather than stress contributing to cancer
    c. stress influences the progression of cancer but not its onset
    d. stress affects the eventual outcome of cancer but not its progress

17. Which of the following is not a valuable psychological component in cancer treatment?
    a. prevention of taste aversions
    b. teaching cognitive and behavioral coping skills
    c. use of thermal biofeedback to control pain
    d. use of guided imagery and relaxation training to control nausea

18. Symptoms of psychopathology such as anxiety, depression, lowered self-esteem and suicidal thoughts
    a. are more likely to occur in homosexual AIDS patients
    b. are more likely to occur in AIDS patients who contracted the disease through blood transfusions
    c. resulting from the social stigma of AIDS may cause further suppression of immune function
    d. are of short duration and therefore do not require professional treatment

19. All of the following are important roles of mental health professionals in meeting the challenge of the AIDS epidemic, except
    a. providing addicts with the means of altering high risk behavior
    b. developing community support for mandatory AIDS testing among high risk populations
    c. counseling homosexual men who engage in high risk sexual behavior
    d. conducting prevention research to find more effective ways to change high risk behaviors

20. Repeatedly dieting and regaining weight, "the yo-yo syndrome"
    a. causes a reduction in metabolic rate
    b. was shown to increase CHD risk in men
    c. both a and b are true
    d. neither a nor b are true

21. Which of the following statements about the role of exercise in weight loss is true?
    a. In one study obese women who walked 30 or more minutes per day lost about 20 pounds in a year while women who walked less failed to lose weight
    b. exercise burns so few calories that heroic efforts are needed for an exercise program to be of benefit to a dieter
    c. exercise produces a compensatory increase in hunger, thereby having little benefit
    d. it is best to exercise strenuously and in private so that the individual will not be interrupted or embarrassed

66

TERMS AND CONCEPTS

Lesson 1
antibodies (154)
antigens (154)
diathesis-stress model (153)
immune system (153)
inflammation (154)
leukocytes (153)
psychoneuroimmunology (154)

Lesson 2
dysmenorrhea (158)
electromyographic biofeedback (157)
estradiol & progesterone (158)
ibuprofen (156)
individual response specificity (156)
migraine headache (156)
premenstrual syndrome (158)
prostaglandins (159)
tension headache (156)
thermal biofeedback (157)

Lesson 3
aerobic exercise (166)
anaerobic exercise (166)
arteriosclerosis (160)
atherosclerosis (161)
cardiovascular disorders (161)
CHD risk factors (162)
coronary heart disease (161)
dietary treatment of hypertension (160)
emotion-focused coping (170)
essential hypertension (160)
problem-focused coping (170)
Type A Behavior (163)

Lesson 4
AIDS (175)
AIDS risks (176)
asthma (172)
coping skills training (174)
immune surveillance theory (173)
pepsin (169)

peptic ulcers (169)
taste aversions (174)

Lesson 5
appetite suppressing drugs (186)
changing antecedents (185)
changing behaviors (185)
changing consequences (185)
eating as oral fixation (181)
external eaters (181)
fat cells (179)
internal eaters (181)
metabolic rate (179)
self-control behavioral treatment (184)
set point (180)
stop center (181)
surgical treatments for obesity (184)
VLCD (182)
yo-yo syndrome (180)

TYING THINGS TOGETHER

1. You be the doctor. If someone comes to you complaining about headaches, what would you do? Make a list of questions you would ask to decide what kind of headache, list the possible methods of treatment for each type and tell which one you would recommend and why.

2. How should research funds be allocated to study the relation of psychological variables and health? Assuming there is more research needed than the available funds will allow, how would you allocate funds among the major disorders in this chapter? Why? Answer these questions and then compare your answers to those of your classmates.

3. A number of themes cut through this chapter: Stress, the diathesis-stress model, behavioral and cognitive therapies, to name a few. Select one of these themes and describe how it is related to health across the variety of disorders in this chapter.

ANSWERS

<u>Lesson 1</u>
1 e
2 a
3 d
4 g
5 b
6 c
7 f

<u>Lesson 2</u>
1 b
2 d
3 a
4 g
5 f
6 i
7 j
8 h
9 e
10 c

<u>Lesson 3</u>
1 d
2 a
3 f
4 h
5 e
6 j
7 g
8 l
9 i
10 k
11 b
12 c

<u>Lesson 4</u>
1 a
2 h
3 c
4 d
5 g

6 f
7 b
8 e

<u>Lesson 5</u>
1 m
2 h
3 c
4 o
5 a
6 i
7 j
8 k
9 f
10 d
11 l
12 g
13 b
14 m
15 e

<u>True-False answers</u>
1 F
2 T
3 F
4 F
5 T
6 F
7 T
8 T
9 T
10 F
11 F
12 T
13 F
14 F
15 F
16 T
17 F
18 T
19 T
20 F
21 T

<u>Multiple-Choice answers</u>
1 c
2 d
3 b
4 b
5 b
6 a
7 a
8 d
9 c
10 a
11 d
12 b
13 d
14 c
15 b
16 a
17 c
18 c
19 b
20 c
21 a

6 Anxiety Disorders

OVERVIEW

The <u>name</u> of this family of disorders tells you something important. Each disorder classified here is included because the primary complaint is anxiety. Anxiety so extreme that it interferes with the individual's ability to function. The chapter introduces anxiety disorders and their historical perspective, then describes the major disorders in this family: Panic disorders, generalized anxiety disorder, phobic disorders and obsessive-compulsive disorder. The major theoretical perspectives on each of these anxiety disorders are described, and the efficacy (effectiveness) of various treatments are evaluated in the discussion of research utilizing them.

One could conceptualize the major ideas you should learn in this chapter as falling into a big table or matrix (in case you're mathematically inclined). Imagine, for a moment, a large sheet of paper covering your entire desk or table. Across the top are columns for the various types of anxiety disorders. Looking down the left side you see (imagine) rows that are labelled characteristics, theoretical perspectives and treatments. Your textbook organized the chapter by describing this imaginary table in words going from left to right across each row (just like your eyes move to read this). As a good student, interested in abnormal psychology, you should try to organize your thinking about this chapter around the imaginary matrix just described.

CHAPTER OUTLINE, LESSONS & LEARNING OBJECTIVES

Lesson 1. Anxiety disorders today and in historical perspective. (213-216)
ANXIETY DISORDERS. (213-214)

Handwritten annotations: Physical - jumpiness, perspiration, sweating, palms, dizziness, diarrhea. Behavioral - Avoidance, clinging dependent behavior, agitated behavior. Cognitive - worrying, nagging, preoccupation. → Mental disorder where prominent feature is anxiety. Formerly called neuroses.

1. Describe the chief features of anxiety and define the term <u>anxiety disorder</u>.

HISTORICAL PERSPECTIVES ON ANXIETY DISORDERS. (214-216)

2. Discuss the historical changes in the classification of anxiety disorders.

Handwritten: Neuroses → anxiety disorder - behavior patterns had biological basis (nervous system). Presently based on similarities in observable behavior & distinct features rather than causation.

Lesson 2. Panic disorder, generalized anxiety disorder, phobic disorders and obsessive-compulsive disorders. (216-225)

PANIC DISORDER. (216-217)

Handwritten: recurrent experience of panic attacks - intense anxiety reactions causing biological reactions (palpitations, dizziness, breathing)

3. Define and describe panic disorder and describe the <u>difference</u> between panic disorder and other forms of anxiety.

Handwritten: more intense than other anxiety problems, with added parts of terror, fear of losing control or dying -impairing

GENERALIZED ANXIETY DISORDER. (217-218)

4. <u>Define</u> and describe generalized anxiety disorder

Handwritten: → Characterized by general feelings of dread + foreboding - heightened states of physiological arousal 6 or 18 features must be present for diagnosis - categories - motor tension, autonomic overarousal, cognitive functioning. - not very impairing

Sim P - persistent, excessive fears of specific objects or situations
Soc P - intense fear of being judged negatively by others
Agora P - fear of places & situations that might be difficult or embarrassing to escape.

PHOBIC DISORDERS. (219-224)

5. Define and describe simple phobia, social phobia and agoraphobia.

OBSESSIVE-COMPULSIVE DISORDER. (224-225)

Ob - recurrent idea that creates anxiety & seems beyond person's control.

6. Define and describe obsessive-compulsive disorder.

characterized by occurrence of obsessional thoughts /compulsions to perform certain actions

Com - irresistible, repetitive urge to perform a certain act

Lesson 3. Theoretical views of anxiety disorders. (225-235)

THEORETICAL VIEWS OF ANXIETY DISORDERS. (225-235)

7. Describe the various theoretical perspectives on the anxiety disorders.

Lesson 4. Treatment of anxiety disorders. (236-242)

TREATMENT OF ANXIETY DISORDERS. (236-242)

Psycho - adaptive behavior

8. Describe the various methods for treating anxiety disorders.

9. Summarize research concerning the effectiveness of various treatment approaches.

Hum - Exist - counseling to get in touch with feelings   Bio - chemotherapy drugs   Learning - Systematic Desensitization
Cognitive - Rational - Emotive cognitive Restructuring.

Mastering Lesson 1: Anxiety disorders today and in historical perspective. (213-216)

Remember that anxiety disorders are characterized by abnormal anxiety that interferes with the ability to function. Specific types of anxiety disorders differ according to the situation that produces it, the intensity and duration of the anxiety and specific things the individual does about it. In mastering this lesson you must try to gain a full appreciation of the problems that abnormal anxiety poses for the individual experiencing it. You must also learn a bit more about how and why disorders were grouped together prior to DSM-III. This is a brief lesson to acquaint you with just a few terms, but it establishes a foundation for the remainder of the chapter.

Match the following terms and concepts with the correct definition or description or explanation.

1. B anxiety
2. A anxiety disorders
3. E etiology cause of disorder
4. D neurosis
5. C psychosis loss contact w/ reality

a. panic disorder, obsessive-compulsive disorder, phobic disorder and generalized anxiety disorder are the major types

b. generalized fear or apprehension about what might happen

c. informal term for severe disorders usually involving loss of contact with reality

d. anxiety disorders were classified here in DSM-II; now an informal term for milder disorders.

e. the causes of a disorder; often forms the basis for classification

7. Psycodynamic
    neuroses
    1. unacceptable impulse into consciousness
    2. fear if they do get to consciousness
    develop them displacement or projection

Learning
    two - factor model
    classical & operant conditioning.

Cognitive
    various thinking patterns
    overprediction of fear,
    oversensitivity to threats
    Irrational Beliefs
    Low Self-Efficacy
    Self-Defeating Thought

Biological
    Genetics - neuroticism
    GABA neurotransmitter is a cause

Mastering Lesson 2. Panic disorder, generalized anxiety disorder, phobic disorders and obsessive-compulsive disorders. (216-225)

In mastering this lesson you must be able to associate the characteristics of each of the types of anxiety disorders with its name. Additionally, you will need to associate specific phobic disorders with their characteristics. You will also need to pay attention to the characteristics that separate each specific disorder from the others (i.e., learn how to tell them apart). As you can see this lesson is much shorter than the number of learning objectives might lead you to think. If you are making a matrix (table) to summarize the chapter, you should fill in the "characteristics" part of your matrix as you complete this lesson. Look at the second exercise in "Tying things together" at the end of this study guide chapter.

Match the following terms and concepts with the correct definition or description or explanation.

1. **B** affects men and women equally often
2. **L** agoraphobia
3. **G** compulsion
4. **A** frequently combines with panic disorder
5. **K** generalized anxiety disorder
6. **C** increases CHD risk
7. **E** likely to abuse alcohol or tranquilizers
8. **H** obsession
9. **M** obsessive-compulsive disorder
10. **I** panic disorder
11. **N** phobia
12. **D** produces avoidance
13. **F** simple phobia
14. **J** social phobia

a. agoraphobia
b. obsessive-compulsive disorder
c. panic disorder
d. phobia
e. social phobic
f. intense irrational fear associated with a specific object or type of situation
g. irresistible, repetitive urge to perform a specific action
h. recurring, uncontrollable thoughts that create anxiety sufficient to interfere with daily life
i. recurring experience of extremely intense bouts of anxiety not tied to environment
j. intense, irrational fear of being judged negatively by others
k. moderate levels of continuous anxiety not attributable to specific environmental event
l. intense, irrational fear of being out in open, busy areas
m. significant distress resulting from repetitive thoughts and/or behaviors
n. persistent fears disportionate to the threat posed by stimuli which elicit them

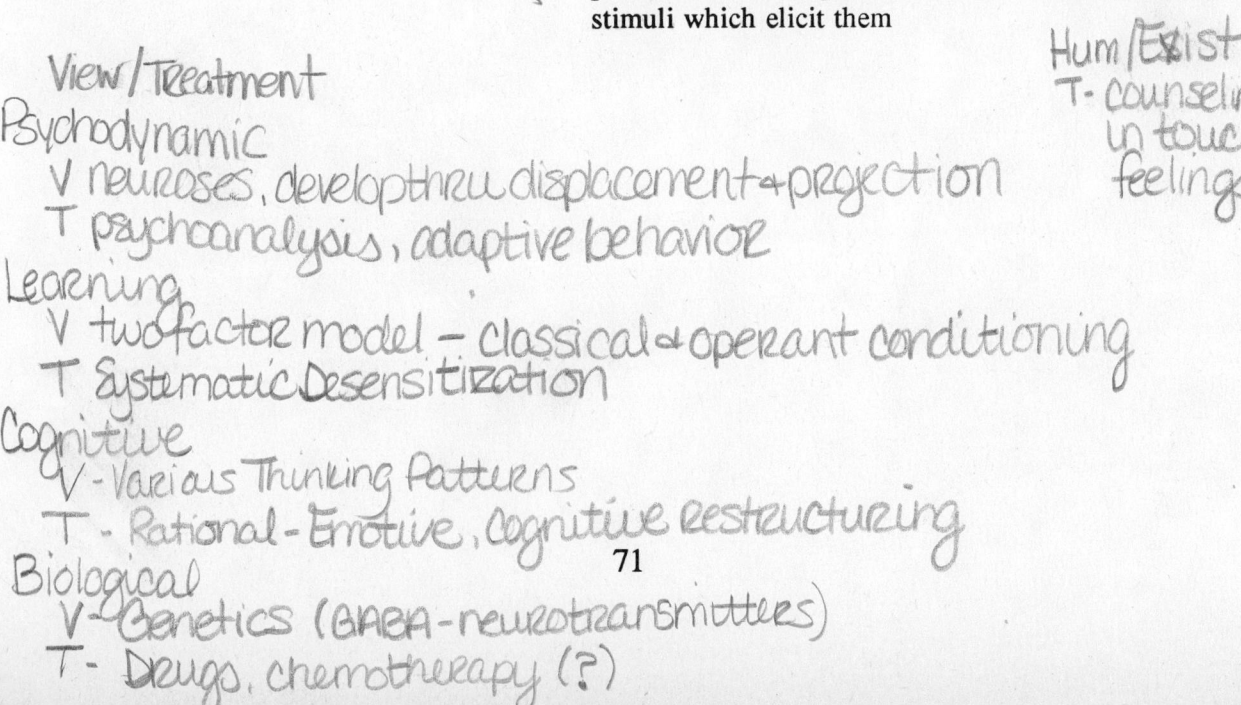

View/Treatment

Psychodynamic
  V neuroses, develop thru displacement + projection
  T psychoanalysis, adaptive behavior

Learning
  V two factor model - classical + operant conditioning
  T Systematic Desensitization

Cognitive
  V - Various Thinking Patterns
  T - Rational-Emotive, Cognitive Restructuring

Biological
  V - Genetics (GABA - neurotransmitters)
  T - Drugs, chemotherapy (?)

Hum/Exist
T- counseling to get in touch with feelings

Mastering Lesson 3. Theoretical views of anxiety disorders. (225-235)

You will discover that this lesson is much more complex than its single learning objective would lead you to expect. It examines the anxiety disorders you just learned about from the psychodynamic, learning, cognitive and biological perspectives. You may find it helpful to quickly review these perspectives in chapter 2 before you continue. Keep in mind that each of these perspectives is trying to account for specific anxiety disorders. In searching for causal relations, they will differ considerably in where they look, but they are all trying to account for the same phenomena. In mastering the information, you will need to associate things in threes: name of the disorder, name of the theoretical perspective and the theoretical explanation. You should also try to understand the logic of how each perspective gets from their causal factor(s) to the characteristics that define the disorder.

If you are making a matrix (table) to summarize the chapter, you should fill in the "theoretical perspectives" part of your matrix as you complete this lesson. Look at the second exercise in "Tying Things Together" at the end of this study guide chapter.

Match the following terms and concepts with the correct definition or description or explanation.

1. M a general biological perspective
2. G classical conditioning
3. F displacement and projection
4. D generalized anxiety disorder-biological perspective
5. L generalized anxiety disorder-learning perspective
6. K generalized anxiety disorder-psychodynamic perspective
7. H hyperventilation
8. R Little Hans
9. O Mowrer's two factor model
10. J obsessive-compulsive disorder-cognitive perspective
11. I obsessive-compulsive disorder-learning perspective
12. B obsessive-compulsive disorder-psychodynamic perspective
13. Q panic disorder-biological perspective
14. C panic disorder-cognitive perspective
15. S panic disorder-psychodynamic perspective
16. E phobicdisorder-cognitive perspective
17. P psychodynamic perspective
18. N self-defeating thoughts
19. A Seligman and Rosenhan's prepared conditioning

a. genetic predisposition to acquire fear of certain things
b. result from reaction formation and fixation
c. vicious cycle resulting from misinterpretation of bodily sensations
d. inadequate inhibition by GABA
e. overprediction of fear leads to avoidance
f. psychodynamic mechanisms for phobias
g. explanation of phobias postulated by the learning perspective
h. enhances fear by reducing blood levels of carbon dioxide
i. reinforced by anxiety reduction
j. irrational beliefs that ritualistic behavior will prevent negative outcomes
k. anxiety from unconscious sources leaks through to consciousness
l. anxiety spreads through stimulus generalization
m. anxiety-related problems tend to run in families
n. in cognitive perspective these serve to heighten and perpetuate anxiety disorders
o. fear of neutral object learned by classical conditioning, maintained by operant avoidance
p. neuroses reflect efforts of repressed impulses to become conscious and the fear that they might
q. thought to be related to serotonin and norepinephrine but direct evidence is lacking
r. Freud's case study in which fear of father was displaced to a horse and became a phobic disorder
s. desperate attempts of ego to repress sexual or aggressive impulses that approach boundaries of consciousness

Mastering Lesson 4. Treatment of anxiety disorders. (236-242)

In this lesson you will encounter descriptions of treatment methods and summaries of some of the research that has attempted to determine treatment efficacy. You will notice that the methods described are organized according to the perspective from which they developed. Therapies which have emerged from the learning and cognitive perspectives are given more attention. This corresponds to the effectiveness of these therapies for the anxiety disorders.

If you are making a matrix (table) to summarize the chapter, you should fill in the "treatment" part of your matrix as you complete this lesson. Look at the second exercise in "Tying Things Together" at the end of this study guide chapter.

Match the following terms and concepts with the correct definition or description or explanation.

1. B biological approaches
2. D cognitive approaches
3. H cognitive therapy
4. E gradual exposure
5. C humanistic-existential therapies
6. G imipramine
7. E learning approaches
8. J psychodynamic approaches
9. I rational-emotive therapy
10. L relaxation training
11. A response prevention
12. M systematicdesensitization
13. K Valium

a. an effective component of behavioral treatment of obsessive-compulsive disorders

b. drugs such as minor tranquilizers, and antidepressants

c. focus on helping people discover and express their talents and feelings

d. family of treatments focusing on altering client's self-defeating thoughts and beliefs

e. family of treatments designed to help people overcome avoidance behavior maintaining phobic disorders

f. treatment approach that has client maintain a state of calmness in the physical presence of successive stimuli in a fear-stimulus hierarchy

g. antidepressant drug has produced some positive results with phobic disorders and mixed results with panic disorder

h. Aaron Beck's cognitive therapy that emphasizes pointing out cognitive errors

i. cognitive therapy developed by Albert Ellis that shows clients how irrational beliefs contribute to anxiety

j. psychoanalysis to free ego from need to control unconscious impulses

k. a minor tranquilizer; the most widely prescribed prescription drug in the world

l. progressive muscle relaxation and biofeedback are two most common methods

m. treatment in which client applies counterconditioning to imagined presence of successive stimuli in a fear-stimulus hierarchy

PRACTICE EXAMS

Exam 1. (true-false).
Indicate whether each of the following statements is **True** or **False**. Question numbers correspond to learning objectives from which the questions were drawn.

1. T Moderate anxiety that does not occur in response to environmental change would be considered abnormal.
2. T Freud's view of neuroses as resulting from threats of anxiety-evoking thoughts emerging into consciousness is still accepted by some clinicians.
3. F Men are about twice as likely to suffer from panic disorder as women.
4. F The difference between generalized anxiety disorder and panic disorder is that the former involves acute, recurring attacks while the latter is usually a chronic condition lasting for at least six months
5. T Phobic disorders are commonly accompanied by extraordinary escape and avoidance behavior.
6. F An obsession is a recurring, irresistible urge to perform an action, commonly in one of two categories: Cleaning or checking.
7. T The cognitive view suggests that anxiety disorders are associated with low self-efficacy expectancies, self-defeating thoughts and inappropriate attributions.
8. T The goal of humanistic-existential therapy for anxiety disorders is to help clients recognize their feelings and use their talents, effectively replacing anxiety with self-confidence and self-acceptance.
9. F Research shows that imipramine may only be effective in the treatment of panic disorders when it is combined with psychodynamic therapy.

Exam 2 (multiple-choice)

Select the single, best answer for each question. Question numbers correspond to learning objectives from which the questions were drawn.

1. Anxiety includes features in which domains?
   a. physical, cognitive and behavioral
   b. physical, emotional and cognitive
   c. emotional, behavioral and cognitive
   d. physical, emotional and behavioral

2. Anxiety disorders were classified as neuroses in DSM-II. This was largely because
   a. of William Cullen's assumption that they had underlying biological causes
   b. the anxiety disorders were grouped with more serious disturbances
   c. of Freud's view that anxiety disorders represented various ways of protecting the ego from anxiety
   d. anxiety disorders were highly resistent to treatment

3. Since many normal people experience a rare bout of panic, in order to be diagnosed as suffering from panic disorder a client must demonstrate at least 4 of 13 physical and cognitive features and
   a. must have a persistent fear lasting at least a month of a recurrence of a panic attack
   b. must have had 4 or more panic attacks in a month
   c. must display excessively high levels of catecholamines
   d. either a or b

4. The diagnosis of generalized anxiety disorder requires
   a. the duration of the anxiety to be at least 3 months
   b. that other possible sources of anxiety be ruled out
   c. the presence of heart palpitations or tachycardia
   d. the presence of feelings of depersonalization

5. The phobic disorder most likely to lead patients to rely on nonphobic companions is
   a. simple phobia
   b. social phobia
   c. acrophobia
   d. agoraphobia

6. The difference between obsessions and delusions is
   a. impossible to determine
   b. that belief in the truth of delusions cannot be shaken
   c. that belief in the truth of obsessions cannot be shaken
   d. that obsessions are behaviors while delusions are thoughts

7. All of the following are explanations of panic disorder except
   a. it is acquired through classical conditioning and maintained by avoidance
   b. results from intense ego activity to prevent sexual or aggressive impulses from reaching consciousness
   c. catastrophic misinterpretations of body sensations that turn into vicious circles
   d. thought to involve serotonin and norepinephrine

8. Analogy: Systematic desensitization is to _____ as imaginary scenes are to environmental stimuli.
   a. psychoanalysis
   b. humanistic-existential therapy
   c. cognitive therapy
   d. gradual exposure

9. Research on the use of cognitive therapies in the treatment of panic disorders has shown that
   a. it was not possible to construct a fear stimulus hierarchy in order to use systematic desensitization
   b. altering client's cognitions about the inevitability of a panic attack was not effective
   c. multifaceted cognitive-behavioral programs eliminate panic attacks in most people
   d. shallow-rapid breathing combined with talking calmly terminates a panic attack

TERMS AND CONCEPTS

TYING THINGS TOGETHER

1. As your text points out, anxiety can be normal or abnormal depending upon its intensity, the appropriateness and its effect on our ability to function. The question is "Where is the point at which anxiety ceases to be normal and must be considered abnormal?" Make a list of the kinds of information you would want to know in order to decide if a client's anxiety should be considered abnormal. Explain how you would use this information to make the decision.

2. Using a **large** sheet of paper, construct a table summarizing the entire chapter. Make columns for each of the types of anxiety disorders. Label the rows "characteristics", "Theoretical Perspectives" and "treatment." You should be able to fit all the important ideas from lessons 2, 3 and 4 into this table. If you are in the electronic era and have a home computer or access to one, you could even do this using one of the spreadsheet programs that are readily available.

3. If you have formed a study group with several classmates, you might wish to each write vignettes, short descriptions of imaginary individuals suffering from different types of anxiety disorders. These could be modeled after the cases presented in the textbook, but edited to eliminate the name of the diagnostic category. Put these on 4 X 6 notecards with the diagnosis on the back. If you can accumulate enough of them, each of you can learn to make diagnoses by reading the vignette, listing the key symptoms, making your diagnosis and then checking the correct diagnosis on the back of the card. If you accumulate these cards over the semester, you can even build them into a game similar to Trivial Pursuit. Become an entrepreneur, publish your game and get rich. Better still, send your cards to WMB or RAH. We will gladly publish your game and get rich.

4. Imagine that you have a loved-one suffering from panic disorder. You have unlimited resources to help this person, but time only permits trying one form of therapy. What kind of therapy would you provide for this individual and why?

ANSWERS

Lesson 1			Lesson 4
1 b	8 h	7 h	1 b
2 a	9 m	8 r	2 d
3 e	10 i	9 o	3 h
4 d	11 n	10 j	4 f
5 c	12 d	11 i	5 c
	13 f	12 b	6 g
	14 j	13 q	7 e
Lesson 2		14 c	8 j
1 b		15 s	9 i
2 l	Lesson 3	16 e	10 l
3 g	1 m	17 p	11 a
4 a	2 g	18 n	12 m
5 k	3 f	19 a	13 k
6 c	4 d		
7 e	5 l		
	6 k		

True-False answers	Multiple-Choice answers
1 T	1 a
2 T	2 c
3 F	3 d
4 F	4 b
5 T	5 c
6 F	6 c
7 T	7 a
8 T	8 d
9 F	9 c

7 Dissociative and Somatoform Disorder

OVERVIEW

If your previous knowledge of abnormal psychology came from movies and television, then the two types of disorders in this chapter should be very familiar. Although dissociative and somatoform disorders are frequently an important element in movies and television programs, these two disorders are, in fact, rather rare. They are much rarer than most of the other disorders about which you will study.

In its first two versions, the Diagnostic and Statistical Manual (DSM) classified dissociative and somatoform disorders as neuroses. The neuroses consisted of those disorders caused by people's attempt to deal with anxiety. Most contemporary analyses of abnormal behavior still discuss dissociative and somatoform disorders together. Although these two disorders show markedly different symptoms, most theoretical viewpoints agree that avoidance of anxiety underlies both of these disorders.

As indicated by the title, this chapter first examines dissociative disorders then somatoform disorders. As usual, the chapter discusses the major diagnostic criteria for each disorder and its major subcategories. This is followed by an examination of the explanations of or the theories for each disorder. While examining competing theories, your chapter discusses important contemporary research on each disorder. You need to pay particular attention to what the researchers did, what they found, and what their results demonstrate. Finally, the examination of the each disorder ends with a brief overview of contemporary treatments for the disorder. As we have mentioned before, whenever you encounter a DSM-III-R disorder, your must learn the diagnostic criteria for that disorder.

CHAPTER OUTLINE, LESSONS & LEARNING OBJECTIVES

Lesson 1. History of dissociative and somatoform disorders. (225-226)
DISSOCIATIVE AND SOMATOFORM DISORDERS (225-226)
1. Explain how the dissociative and somatoform disorders differ from the anxiety disorders in terms of the theorized role of anxiety.
2. Describe the historical changes in the classification of these diagnostic classes.

Lesson 2. Dissociative disorders. (226-238)
THE DISSOCIATIVE DISORDERS. (226-238)
3. Describe the symptoms of the dissociative disorders.
4. Describe multiple personality disorder.
5. Describe psychogenic amnesia and distinguish it from other amnesias.
6. Describe psychogenic fugue.
7. Describe the depersonalization disorder.

8. Explain why some clinicians believe the depersonalization disorder is not a dissociative disorder.
9. Explain how each major theory accounts for the occurrence of dissociative disorders.
10. What were the procedure, results, and significance of the Spanos study, which was inspired by the Hillside Strangler.
11. Describe the major treatments for dissociative disorders.

Lesson 3. Somatoform disorders. (238-244)
SOMATOFORM DISORDERS. (238-244)
12. Describe the major symptoms of the three major somatoform disorders: conversion disorder, hypochondriasis, and somatization disorder.
13. Explain how each major theory accounts for the occurrence of somatoform disorders.
14. Explain how a somatoform disorder differs from malingering.
15. Describe the symptoms of Munchausen syndrome and theories for its occurrence.

Mastering Lesson 1. History of dissociative and somatoform disorders. (225-226)

This lesson is brief and straight forward. You need to memorize brief descriptions of two abnormal behaviors, dissociative and somatoform disorders. You will also need to remember persons suffering from anxiety disorders experience or feel anxiety as a part of their problems. On the other hand, persons suffering from dissociative and somatoform disorders do not usually experience or feel anxiety even though these disorders may represent attempts to avoid anxiety. Finally, you need to know about differences between DSM-II and DSM-III-R. DSM-II grouped anxiety, dissociative, and somatoform disorders together under the classification of neurosis because classifications were based upon theoretical assumption, primarily psychodynamic. DSM-III-R does not group anxiety, dissociative, and somatoform disorders together because classifications are now based upon observable patterns of behavior.

Match the following terms and concepts with the correct definition or description or explanation.

1. C anxiety disorders
2. E dissociative disorders
3. B DSM-II
4. A DSM-III-R
5. D somatoform disorders

a. classification system based upon patterns of observable behavior
b. classification system based upon psychodynamic theory
c. disorders in which anxiety is directly expressed in symptoms
d. disorders showing physical symptoms without organic basis or anxiety
e. disorders showing psychological difficulties without manifest anxiety

Mastering Lesson 2. Dissociative disorders. (226-238)

This section examines the four subclassifications of dissociative disorders, multiple personality, psychogenic amnesia (which has four sub-types), psychogenic fugue, and depersonalization disorder. You will need to know the diagnostic criteria for these disorders and their subtypes. You will need to be able to differentiate these disorders.   The two most difficult disorders to differentiate are psychogenic amnesia and psychogenic fugue. Try to remember that "fugue" means "flight," that is, the "fugue" of psychogenic fugue literally means to run away.

Two major theoretical analyses of dissociative disorders are discussed in you text. Both of these approaches emphasize that the symptoms appear as the person attempts to avoid anxiety because it is unpleasant. The psychodynamic approach differs from the learning-cognitive approach by assuming that there is a complex underlying psychological structure of id, ego, and superego. The learning-cognitive approach puts more emphasis on modeling and the direct consequences of behaving abnormally.

This lesson ends with a discussion of treatment. Very little is known about how to treat dissociative disorders because they are so rare. That is, very few people have received any kind of treatment for dissociative disorders.

Match the following terms and concepts with the correct definition or description or explanation.

1. A continuous amnesia *problem/trauma*
2. M depersonalization disorder
3. G derealization
4. F dissociative disorder
5. D generalized amnesia *entire*
6. I Learning-Cognitive perspective
 7. C localized amnesia *tion*
8. J malingering
9. N multiple personality
10. H Nicholas Spanos
11. E Psychodynamic perspective
12. B psychogenic amnesia
13. L psychogenic fugue
14. K selective amnesia *for parts*

a. a continuing inability to remember events after a trauma
b. a sudden loss of memory not attributable to physical problems
c. amnesia for specific details of a guilt arousing event
d. an inability to remember any of the details of one's life
e. ego avoids memories of trauma through repression and dissociation
f. identity, memory, or consciousness are no longer integrated
g. marked changes in the perception of one's surroundings or time
h. multiple personality may result from role-playing to social cues
i. observation of dissociative disorders models ways to avoid anxiety
j. pretending to be amnesiac to escape responsibility
k. psychogenic amnesia for a fixed period of time following a trauma
l. psychogenic amnesia with a change of location and a new identity
m. recurrent feelings of detachment from one's body
n. two distinct personalities take control over a person's behavior

81

Mastering Lesson 3. Somatoform disorders. (238-244)

The analysis of somatoform disorders involves learning the diagnostic criteria for conversion disorder, hypochondriasis, and somatization disorder. We find that students often confuse "somatoform" and "somatization." The first is the general classification; the second is a particular type. Diagnoses of these disorders requires paying attention to numbers, age and number of symptoms presented. For example, the somatization disorder is diagnosed only if 13 different symptoms are present and those symptoms come from 6 different categories of 35 symptoms. The two major explanations of somatoform disorders, psychodynamic and learning, your text examines in detail. The chapter ends with a very brief analysis of treatment.

Match the following terms and concepts with the correct definition or description or explanation.

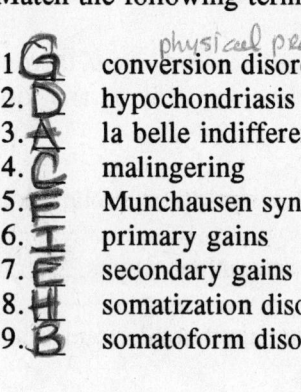

physical problems

1. G conversion disorder
2. D hypochondriasis
3. A la belle indifference
4. C malingering
5. E Munchausen syndrome
6. I primary gains
7. E secondary gains
8. H somatization disorder
9. B somatoform disorder

a. an apparent lack of concern about a conversion disorder symptom
b. complaints of physical symptoms without organic abnormalities
c. consciously and deliberately faking symptoms to obtain rewards
d. excessive fear of illness without medical foundation
e. external rewards for symptomatic behavior
f. factitious disorder
g. loss of sensory or motor functions without physical cause
h. multiple and persistent physical complaints without physical cause
i. psychodynamic term for relief from unconscious conflicts

PRACTICE EXAM

Exam 1. (true-false)

Indicate whether each of the following statements is **True** or **False**. Question numbers correspond to learning objectives from which the questions were drawn.

1. T Individuals suffering from somatoform disorders are frequently unconcerned about their problems.
2. F DSM-II is more behavioral in its orientation than DSM-III-R.
3. T Psychogenic depersonalization is one of the dissociative disorders.
4. T More than 500 cases of multiple personality have been analyzed.
5. F Continuous amnesia is the most common form of psychogenic amnesia. *localized - T*
6. F Persons malingering and pretending a psychogenic fugue are easily detected.
7. T Depersonalization may involve derealization.
8. F Depersonalization disorder always lowers a person's anxiety levels.
9. F Most children who suffer child abuse develop dissociative disorders. *few*
10. T Most normal people will reveal a second personality if asked to do so under hypnosis.

82

11. **F** Derealization therapy is very effective in treating multiple personality.
12. **T** Hypochondriasis does <u>not</u> involve the presence of any physical ailments.
13. **F** Learning theorist's assume that conversion disorders always involve faking.
14. **F** Malingering is short-term somatization disorder of frequent occurrence.
15. **T** With factitious disorders, there is no obvious secondary gain.

Exam 2 (multiple-choice)

Select the single, best answer for each question. Question numbers correspond to learning objectives from which the questions were drawn.

1. In which of the following disorders, would a person feel high levels of anxiety and dread?
   - a. anxiety disorder
   - b. dissociative disorder
   - c. multiple personality
   - d. somatoform disorder

2. DSM-II grouped anxiety, dissociative, and somatoform disorders together because
   - a. the learning perspective assumes that all of these disorders are due to anxiety
   - b. the psychodynamic perspective assumes that all of these disorders are due to anxiety
   - c. the cognitive perspective assumes that all of these disorders result from a lack of meaning in one's life
   - d. the psychodynamic perspective assumes that all of these disorders result from either heterophobia or homophobia

3. Dissociative disorders involve a disintegration of the unity of
   - a. affect but not memory
   - b. identity but not affect
   - c. memory but not identity
   - d. consciousness but not memory

4. The individual personalities of a person suffering from a multiple personality disorder are
   - a. usually schizophrenic
   - b. present at the same time
   - c. well integrated
   - d. always aware of each other

5. If a person is unable to remember anything about the week after their father died, they have what type of psychogenic amnesia?
   - a. continuous amnesia
   - b. generalized amnesia
   - c. localized amnesia
   - d. selective amnesia

6. Psychogenic fugue involves all but one of the following. Which of the following symptoms is <u>not</u> a symptom of a psychogenic fugue?
   a. loss of memory for the past
   b. assumption of a new identity
   c. sudden travel from home
   d. a schizophrenic new personality

7. DSM-III-R suggests that the majority of young adults will encounter the feeling that they are detached from their bodies or minds. They are <u>not</u> diagnosed as having a depersonalization disorder because
   a. they are too young to be diagnosed
   b. depersonalization only involves emotions
   c. the detachment is only temporary
   d. young adults are never disturbed by the experience

8. Depersonalization disorder differs from the other dissociative disorders in that depersonalization
   a. involves no memory disturbance
   b. produces little distress for the person
   c. symptoms are long lasting
   d. occurs more frequently in females

9. The learning-cognitive perspective of dissociative disorders suggests that
   a. people generally enjoying thinking about unpleasant events
   b. children are too young to learn maladaptive behaviors
   c. people may be reinforced for maladaptive behaviors
   d. most people have little or no idea what a multiple personality is

10. Nicholas Spanos conducted an experiment modeled after the interrogation of the Hillside strangler, Kenneth Bianchi. Spanos used three groups
    a. his control group spontaneously reported a second self 35% of the time
    b. his hidden-part condition refused to answer the Bianchi question
    c. 81% of his Bianchi condition revealed a second self when asked
    d. his subjects who revealed a second self remembered they did so later

11. Which dissociative disorder is most subject to treatment?
    a. depersonalization
    b. multiple personality
    c. psychogenic amnesia
    d. psychogenic fugue

12. Diagnosis of a conversion disorder
    a. requires the presence of multiple physical symptoms
    b. always involves a loss of sexual functioning
    c. is relatively easy and seldom in error
    d. may be made in the case of a false pregnancy

13. According to some learning theorists, hypochondriasis is a form of
    a. schizophrenia
    b. manic-depressive disorder
    c. multiple personality
    d. obsessive-compulsive disorder

14. Persons suffering from conversion disorder differ from persons malingering in that persons suffering from a conversion disorder
    a. are not consciously inventing symptoms
    b. are more likely to be blind
    c. have more medically accurate symptoms
    d. receive no secondary gains

15. Factitious disorders
    a. are more frequent among racial minorities
    b. have an obvious primary gain
    c. involve maladaptive behavior
    d. seldom involve deliberate faking

TERMS AND CONCEPTS

Lesson 1
anxiety disorders (225)
dissociative disorders (225)
DSM-II (226)
DSM-III-R (226)
somatoform disorders (225)

Lesson 2
continuous amnesia (230)
depersonalization disorder (231)
derealization (231)
dissociative disorder (226)
generalized amnesia (230)
Learning-Cognitive perspective (235)
localized amnesia (230)
malingering (230)
multiple personality (226)
Nicholas Spanos (236)
Psychodynamic perspective (235)
psychogenic amnesia (229)
psychogenic fugue (230)
selective amnesia (230)

Lesson 3
conversion disorder (238)
hypochondriasis (239)
la belle indifference (238)
malingering (243)
Munchausen syndrome (244)
primary gains (241)
secondary gains (241)
somatization disorder (240)
somatoform disorder (238)

TYING THINGS TOGETHER

1. In light of the Spanos study, what special difficulties exist in accurately diagnosing multiple personalities? What steps might a clinician take to avoid these problems?

2. Using the concept of secondary gain, explain why the occurrence of conversion disorders may in fact be greater among women than men.

ANSWERS

Lesson 1
1 c
2 e
3 b
4 a
5 d

Lesson 2
1 a
2 m
3 g
4 f
5 d
6 i
7 c
8 j
9 n
10 h
11 e
12 b
13 l
14 k

Lesson 3
1 g
2 d
3 a
4 c
5 f
6 i
7 e
8 h
9 b

True-False answers
1 T
2 F
3 F
4 F
5 F
6 F
7 T
8 F
9 F
10 T
11 F
12 T
13 F
14 F
15 T

Multiple-Choice answers
1 a
2 b
3 b
4 c
5 d
6 d
7 c
8 a
9 c
10 c
11 b
12 d
13 d
14 a
15 c

8 Mood Disorders and Suicide

OVERVIEW

This chapter covers mood disorders, one of which, depression, is the "common cold" of abnormal psychology. The relatively high frequency of the mood disorders makes understanding them important and has two consequences. The first is that a great deal is known about them. Therefore, the chapter on mood disorders is long, although there are only four mood disorders. The second is that there has been considerable effort to find a cure for this "common cold". Thus, there are numerous and complex theories and treatments for mood disorders.

The chapter begins with the description of the characteristics of the mood disorders. There are four major mood disorders, major depression, dysthymia, bipolar disorder, and cyclothymia. Major depression is broken down into four subtypes, seasonal affective disorder, endogenous depression, reactive depression, and postpartum depression.

A discussion of the major theories follows the discussion of the characteristics or diagnostic criteria of the mood disorders. Theories of mood disorders can be grouped into two large categories the psychological and the biological. Psychodynamic theory, humanist-existential, learning, and cognitive compose the psychological theories. Genetic and biochemical compose the biological theories. Again, because of the importance or mood disorders, every theoretical perspective has a lot to say about them.

The chapter continues with a discussion of treatments for the mood disorders. These treatments can be grouped in the same way the theories are grouped. The chapter ends with a discussion of suicide and its treatment. Suicide, although not one of the DSM-III-R categories, is usually combined with a discussion of depression. This reflects the importance of depression in producing suicide. An understanding of suicide requires an understanding of depression.

CHAPTER OUTLINE, LESSONS & LEARNING OBJECTIVES

Lesson 1. Defining the mood disorder. (250-259)
MOOD DISORDERS. (250) ↗ *characterized by disturbances in mood that are serious enough to impair daily functioning.*
1. Define and identify the mood disorders. → *major depression & dysthymia, bipolar, & cyclothymia*
MAJOR DEPRESSION. (250-257)
2. Describe the difference between normal and abnormal depressed mood.
3. Describe the characteristics of major depression. *↳ severe, last long time, affect daily functioning.*

↳ Δmood, crying, unmotivated, low social participation,
loss of interest, Δsleeping habits, Δappetite, func.
less effectively, dif. concentrate, think neg.
lack self-esteem, think of death or suicide.
(Δ's- emotional states, motivation, functioning + motor behavior + cognition)

R-psychologically based

E-biologically based, char. by physical features of depression

4. Describe the course of major depression. *makes it more difficult to ear*

5. Explain the role of stress in depression and the frequency of major depression. *report more stressful events S+D - correlational not experimental*

6. Describe seasonal affective disorder. *Fatigue, excessive sleep, carbo craving, weight g*

7. Explain the difference between reactive and endogenous depression. *genetic + women - men*

8. Describe postpartum depression. *severe mood changes after childbirth. At risk - 1st time m single mom, lack social support, women more optimistic about the baby.*

DYSTHYMIA. (257)

✳ **9.** Describe the characteristics of dysthymia and explain how it differs from major depression. *not severly depressed, occurs more days than not*

BIPOLAR DISORDER. (257-259)

10. Describe the characteristics of bipolar disorder. *severe mood swings (manias → depression).*

11. Describe the feature of a manic episode. *emotional roller coaster, pressured speech M+W = Rapid flight of ideas, multiple tasks, hallucinations, delusions*

CYCLOTHYMIA. (259)

people may be depressed when learn to view themselves as helpless to control reinforcement in environment + to ▲ life for better. (Situational factors) Result from exposure to uncontrollable situations. Attry - when disappointments or failures occur, we may explain in various ways (Internal/ex, global/specific, stable/unstable)

✳ **12.** Describe the characteristics of cyclothymia and explain how it differs from bipolar disorder. *chronic, cyclical pattern of mood swings, at least 2 yrs duration, Hypomanic*

C is milder form of B.D. - boundaries not clearly established.

Lesson 2. Theories of the origins of the mood disorders. (260-274)

THEORETICAL PERSPECTIVES. (260-274)

13. Discuss the psychodynamic explanation for the mood disorders. *d. rep. anger directed inward at self, mourning-pathological mourning - occurs in people w/ ambivalent f to preserve lost object - introjects rep*

14. Discuss behavioral explanation for the mood disorders especially the relationship between reinforcement and depression. *focusing model - attentional process favor-develops Dep. Results - behave - too little reinforcement too little reinf. → strive for more reinf. → inactivity for reinf. → dep*

MZ - 40% DZ 11% - Dep. disorders

15. Discuss Beck's cognitive theory of depression and the reformulated helplessness (attributional) theory. *Cog triad of depr. → Schemas = views - View oneself, - View environment, - view future. All-nothing thinking, overgeneralization mental filter, Disqual. +, jump conclusions, Magnif+min, Emo reasoning, shou labeling, mislabeling pers*

D ST - oral steroid → no cortisol - somett 40%-50% sensitivity +DST - help confirm a depressive disorder - DST - not contradict presence of dep. limits - may pick up effects of other drugs + not dep. predict response to antidep.

16. Discuss the evidence which suggests that there is genetic disposition to depression.

17. Discuss biochemical explanations for depression, particularly the catecholamine hypothesis. *Dep. from deficiencies in norepinepheine, excessive - manic.*

18. Discuss how the dexamethasone suppression test is used to diagnose depression.

19. Discuss the evidence that creative genius is related to mood disorder.

Lesson 3. Treating the mood disorders and suicide. (274-286)

TREATMENT. (274-281)

dep uncover feelings of lost object.

20. Describe the psychodynamic treatment for mood disorders.

helps dep clients identify distorted, self-defeating thoughts + beliefs + substitute more rational ones. 16-20 weekly sessions

21. Describe Lewinsohn's *Coping with Depression Course* as a behavioral treatment for mood disorders. *helps dep. clients get relaxation skills, + partic in pleasant activities acquire social skills to get reinforcement from others. No side* *people - students, homework, lectures, activi*

22. Describe Beck's cognitive therapy for the treatment of mood disorders. *affect neurotransmitters in brain interfere w/ reuptake, conc ↑*

23. Describe the use of antidepressants, tricyclics and MAO inhibitor drugs as treatments.

24. Describe the use of lithium as a treatment for bipolar disorder.

25. Discuss the pros and cons of using ECT as a treatment for depression.

SUICIDE. (281-286)

TANYA WAS BITCHIN YOU BACKED OUT ON HER

26. Discuss the incidence of suicide. *1/4 mil attempt, 30,000 die. White males most, black f least, elderly*

27. Briefly discuss theories of suicide.

28. Describe ways to prevent suicide.

27. *Psychodynamic - suicidal people seek to destroy self, but vent murderous rage against love object internalized*
Existential + Humanistic - perception life is meaningless + lacks a purpose + hope
Sociocultural - alienation in present-day society,
Learning - reinforcing effects of prior suicide threats + attempts + to effects of stress.
combined w/ lack of coping skills.
Social + Cognitive - suicide motivated by + outcome expectancies. (missed, eulogized)
→ modeling in society,

28. *Signs - hopelessness, loss pleasure, interest, reactivity. moodswings, fewer friendship adolescence.*

Psy - anger directed inward, talk about feelings
Beh - too little reinforcement, get reinforcement, teach coping skills
Cog - triad of depression
Biochem - deficiences in neurotranstr, antidepressants, tricyclics MAO

Mastering Lesson 1. Defining the mood disorders. (250-259)

This first lesson covers the diagnostic criteria for the four major mood disorders and the four subtypes of major depression. You will need to know the material summarized by Table 8.1 in your text very well to differentiate major depression, dysthymia, bipolar disorder, and cyclothymia. However, do not rely on this table alone. Important information that will help you distinguish these disorders is contained in discussion in your text. Because major depression is the most important of these four disorders, you should know its diagnostic features, which are summarized in Table 8.3 in your text. The four subtypes of major depression, seasonal affective disorder, endogenous depression, reactive depression, and postpartum depression are not neatly summarized in a table. Therefore, you should make up a summary table for yourself.

As with many other disorder, distinguishing the normal from the abnormal can be difficult. Considering how common both normal and abnormal depression are, distinguishing them becomes more important.

Finally, an important part of the analysis of the mood disorders is an understanding of its demographics. That is, it is important to know the who, what, and when of the major disorder and the subtypes. Sex, age, social support, and environmental factors are all related to developing a mood disorder, in general, as well as a specific category.

Match the following terms and concepts with the correct definition or description or explanation.

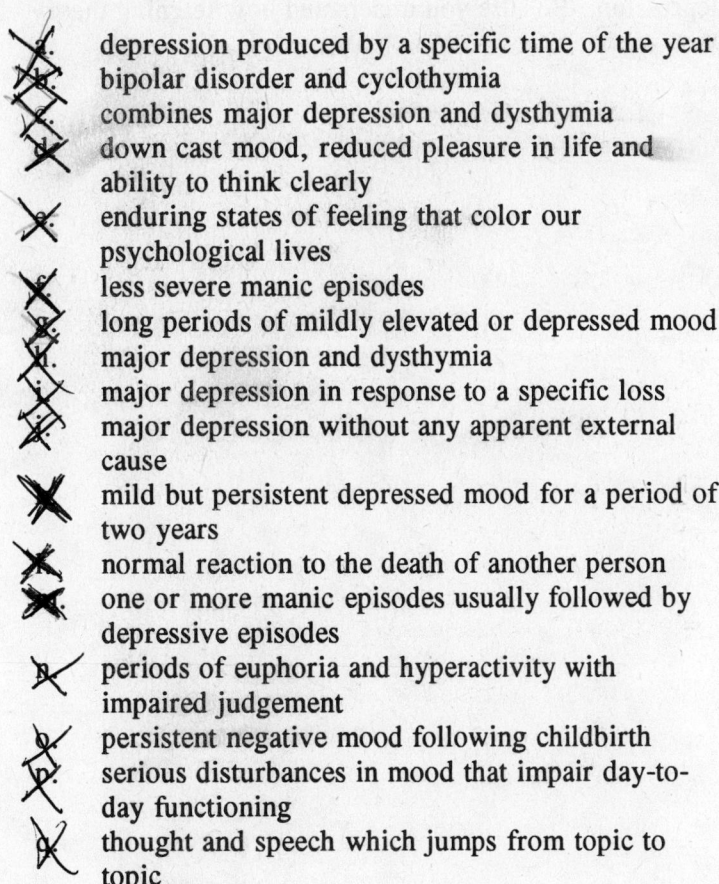

1. L   bereavement
2. M   bipolar disorder
3. G   cyclothymia
4. C   double depression
5. K   dysthymia
6. J   endogenous depression
7. F   hypo-manic episodes
8. D   major depression
9. N   manic episodes
10. P   mood disorders
11. E   moods
12. O   postpartum depression
13. Q   rapid flight of ideas
14. I   reactive depression
15. A   seasonal affective disorder
16. B   the bipolar disorders
17. H   the depressive disorders

a. depression produced by a specific time of the year
b. bipolar disorder and cyclothymia
c. combines major depression and dysthymia
d. down cast mood, reduced pleasure in life and ability to think clearly
e. enduring states of feeling that color our psychological lives
f. less severe manic episodes
g. long periods of mildly elevated or depressed mood
h. major depression and dysthymia
i. major depression in response to a specific loss
j. major depression without any apparent external cause
k. mild but persistent depressed mood for a period of two years
l. normal reaction to the death of another person
m. one or more manic episodes usually followed by depressive episodes
n. periods of euphoria and hyperactivity with impaired judgement
o. persistent negative mood following childbirth
p. serious disturbances in mood that impair day-to-day functioning
q. thought and speech which jumps from topic to topic

91

Mastering Lesson 2. Theories of the origins of the mood disorders (260-274)

There are six major theories of mood disorders, Psychodynamic, humanist-existential, learning, cognitive, genetic and biochemical. The Psychodynamic and humanist-existential are the easiest. Your text provides short and simple presentations of them. The most difficult theories to understand are the cognitive and biochemical theories. The cognitive theory is difficult because it is composed of many parts. There is the cognitive triad of depression (Table 8.4 of your text), the ten cognitive distortions, the automatic thoughts associated with depression and anxiety (Table 8.5 of your text), and Seligman's attributional style model to learn. The individual pieces are not hard to understand or learn but there are a lot of them.

The processes described by the biochemical theory are just plain complex, particularly the action of MAO inhibitors. The best way to really learn this is to make a diagram of the process. Step 1, catecholamine are in synapses and stimulating neurons. Step 2, monoamine oxidase breaks down catecholamine. This prevents them from stimulating neurons. Step 3, MAO inhibitors bind or join with monoamine oxidase (MAO) to prevent (another word for inhibit) from breaking down the catecholamine. Step 4, if MAO inhibitors are present, MAO is not present and catecholamine levels stay high. If MAO inhibitors are absent, MAO is present and catecholamine levels are reduced. Go over this information repeatedly, until you can walk down the street, chew gum, and describe the process, all at the same time. Because understanding how MAO inhibitors work requires one to read carefully and pay attention to detail, asking test questions about them is a great favorite of instructors. At least, we ask exam questions which cover this process in detail.

Finally, do not be mislead by the moderate level of complexity of the learning theory of depression. Be sure you understand how learning theory views depression as a vicious circle phenomenon.

Match the following terms and concepts with the correct definition or description or explanation.

1. E Aaron Beck
2. U ambivalent
3. P automatic thoughts
4. B catastrophizing
5. M catecholamine hypothesis
6. L cognitive distortions
7. T Cognitive theory
8. N cognitive-specificity hypothesis
9. H Humanist-Existential Theory
10. A Interactional theory
11. Q introject
12. F learned helplessness theory
13. I Learning Theory
14. D musterbation
15. S negative view of oneself
16. R negative view of the environment
17. V negative view of the future
18. G Psychodynamic theory
19. K reformulated helplessness theory
20. C selective abstraction
21. J self-focusing model
22. O tricyclics and monamine oxidase inhibitors

a. acting depressed elicits subtle negative reactions from loved ones
b. cognitive distortion exaggerating the importance of negative events
c. cognitive distortion in which only negative features are remembered
d. cognitive distortion producing unrealistic self expectations
e. cognitive theory of depression
f. depressed people believe they are unable to control their environment
g. depression is due to anger against the self
h. depression is due to disruption in personality identity due to a loss
i. depression is due to inadequate levels of reinforcement
j. depression is due to lowered self-esteem following a loss
k. depression is due to the types of attributions a person makes
l. depression is due to the cognitive triad of depression
m. depression results from deficient levels of norepinephrine
n. different disorders are characterized by different automatic thoughts
o. drugs which increase norepinephrine levels in the brain
p. habitual thoughts are accepted without analysis as facts
q. incorporating another person into one's self
r. perceiving demands or obstacles that are impossible to overcome
s. perceiving oneself as worthless, deficient, unlovable
t. specific errors in thinking that can lead to depression
u. strongly negative and strongly positive
v. the expectation of continuing failure and unending hardship

93

Mastering Lesson 3. Treating the mood disorders and suicide. (274-281)

If you fully understand the theories of mood disorder from Lesson 2, understanding the treatments will be relatively straightforward and easy. **Do not** try this lesson unless you fully understand the material of Lesson 2. You should pay particular attention to information about the effectiveness of the various treatments because the frequency of the mood disorders makes an analysis of their effectiveness possible.

Psychoanalytic and humanist-existential treatments are straight forward. Learning theory or behavioral treatment as exemplified by Lewinsohn's *Coping with Depression Course* will be best understood by a careful reading of the case study presented in your text.

Although understanding cognitive theory is difficult due to the large number of concepts, cognitive therapy in the abstract is relatively easy. Cognitive therapy involves changing how people think about things. Exactly what kind of changes in thinking cognitive therapy produces is summarized in Table 8.6 of your text, "Cognitive Distortion and Rational Responses." Read through this table carefully without necessarily trying to memorize its contents. Make sure you understand why the thought in the "Automatic Thought" column is distorted and an example of the type of cognitive distortion in the middle column. Then, go to the right hand column, and explain to yourself why that response is more rational.

Your text discusses three biological approaches to therapy, antidepressant drug therapy, lithium therapy, and ECT. Understanding antidepressant drug therapies is totally dependent on understanding the biochemical theories of mood disorders. Once, you understand the theory the therapy will be understood and learned easily. You encountered no theory for lithium therapy or ECT in Lesson 2 because both treatments lack a coherent explanation for their effectiveness. Therefore, you will need to pay particular attention to the limiting conditions under which lithium and ECT may work. With all of the biological treatments, side effects are a major concern.

Finally, one of the major antecedents to suicide is depression. Therefore, suicide is discussed in this chapter. The analysis of suicide focuses on the prediction of its occurrence based upon demographic variables, such as age and sex, environmental conditions, and the presence of mood disorders.

Match the following terms and concepts with the correct definition or description or explanation.

1. H antidepressant drug therapy
2. D behavioral treatment
3. F cognitive therapy
4. C Coping with Depression Course
5. A electroconvulsive therapy
6. E humanist-existential treatment
7. G lithium therapy
8. B psychodynamic treatment

a. administering electrical current to the head
b. attempts to uncover ambivalent feelings toward lost object
c. behavioral treatment of relaxation, pleasant activity, and social skills
d. focuses on directly modifying depressive behaviors
e. focuses on finding meaning through self-actualization
f. identifies distorted thoughts and substitutes rational ones
g. ingestion of lithium carbonate to control bipolar disorder
h. uses tricyclics and monoamine oxidase inhibitors

PRACTICE EXAM

Exam 1. (true-false)

Indicate whether each of the following statements is **True** or **False**. Question numbers correspond to learning objectives from which the questions were drawn.

1. F   There are three major categories of mood disorders.
2. F   Normal depression does not typically interfere with our ability to function.
3. F   Persons suffering from major depression are always listless.
4. T   Most persons suffering one episode of major depression will experience another one.
5. T   Women are more likely to experience a major depression than men.
6. T   The symptoms of a seasonal affective disorder are very similar to those of a major depression.
7. F   Reactive depression is thought to be biological in nature.
8. F   Postpartum depression is an extremely rare problem.
9. T   Dysthymia is milder than major depression.
10. F   Persons suffering from bipolar disorder never attempt suicide in the manic phase.
11. F   Manic episodes begin slowly and develop gradually.
12. T   Cyclothymia may develop into bipolar disorder.
13. F   Research evidence clearly shows that repressed anger toward the dead turned inward produces depression.
14. T   According to learning theory, depression results from too little reinforcement from one's environment.
15. F   "I am going to be injured" is a common automatic thought associated with depression.
16. F   Genetics plays a major role in explaining mood disorders.
17. F   MAO inhibitors suppress catecholamine activity.
18. T   The dexamethasone suppression test finds many false positives.
19. F   Highly creative people are generally insane.
20. F   Traditional psychoanalysis for depression requires a few weeks.
21. F   The *Coping with Depression Course* is based upon psychoanalytic principles.
22. F   Cognitive therapy and behavior therapy both involve a relatively long period of treatment.
23. F   Lithium is used exclusively to treat major depression.
24. F   MAO inhibitors are used to treat bipolar disorder.
25. F   Electroconvulsive therapy is the treatment of first choice for depression.
26. T   More males "succeed" in committing suicide than females.
27. F   Suicide in a clear sign of insanity.
28. F   Most people who commit suicide give no warning.

<u>Exam 2 (multiple-choice)</u>

Select the single, best answer for each question. Question numbers correspond to learning objectives from which the questions were drawn.

1. There are _____ types of mood disorders.
    a. 2
    b. 4
    c. 5
    d. 6

2. Which of <u>the following</u> would be typical of a normally depressed person?
    a. depressed mood passes quickly
    b. large decrease in physical activity
    c. recurrent thoughts of suicide
    d. faulty perceptions of reality

3. Which of the following is a diagnostic feature of major depression?
    a. short periods of depressed mood
    b. deliberate increase in weight
    c. daily inability to sleep
    d. repetitive and stereotyped motoric activity

C

4. A person who overcomes an episode of major depression
    a. is unlikely to have another one within a two year period
    b. has a 50% chance of having one in two years
    c. is more likely to have another episode the longer they go without one
    d. is more likely to develop schizophrenia than a person who has never had an episode

B

5. Which of the following groups has the highest rate of depression?
    a. women who have never been married
    b. married men
    c. married women
    d. men who have recently been divorced

C

6. Which of the following persons is most likely to suffer from a seasonal affective disorder?
    a. an adolescent female
    b. a middle-aged male
    c. a retired male
    d. a middle-aged female

A

7. A depression produced by a precipitating event is what kind of depression?
    a. endogenous
    b. major
    c. precipitated
    d. reactive

D

96

8. Which of the following decreases the likelihood a mother will have postpartum depression?

A
   a. general optimism about life
   b. optimism about one's baby
   c. being single
   d. a first pregnancy

9. How does dysthymia differ from major depression?

D
   a. Major depression lasts longer than dysthymia
   b. Dysthymia is characterized by mild manic episodes
   c. Major depression functions as part of a person's personality
   d. Dysthymia's mood alteration is less severe

10. Bipolar disorder is characterized by

B
   a. one or two years of mania followed by a year or two of depression
   b. short manic episodes followed by longer depressive episodes
   c. short depressive episodes followed by longer manic episodes
   d. four or five manic-depressive cycles per year

11. Which of the following is <u>not</u> one of the characteristics of a manic episode?

D
   a. pressured speech
   b. violent outbursts
   c. rapid flight of ideas
   d. hallucinations

12. Bipolar disorder is characterized by _____ manic episodes and _____ depressive episodes than cyclothymia.

D
   a. milder, milder
   b. milder, stronger
   c. stronger, milder
   d. stronger, stronger

13. According to Psychoanalytic theory, the _____ is the dominant part of the personality during depressive episodes of bipolar disorder.

C
   a. conscious
   b. ego
   c. id
   d. superego

14. Learning theory suggests that inactivity and depressed feeling of a depressive episode usually produces

C
   a. little change in the environment which maintains a stable level of depression
   b. little response by one's family and thus acting out for attention
   c. a further decrease in reinforcement and increasingly severe depression
   d. sympathy and understanding from one's family lessening the depression

97

15. Which of the following is not one of the elements of Aaron Beck's cognitive triad of depression?
    a. negative view of others
    b. negative view of oneself
    c. negative view of the environment
    d. negative view of the future

16. MZ twins show _____ concordance for major depression and _____ concordance for bipolar disorder than DZ twins.
    a. higher, higher
    b. higher, lower
    c. lower, higher
    d. lower, lower

17. According to the catecholamine hypothesis, high levels of epinephrine produce
    a. manic episodes
    b. depressive episodes
    c. dysthymia
    d. a bipolar shift

18. In the dexamethasone test for depression, depression is indicated by
    a. high levels of cortisol
    b. low levels of cortisol
    c. low levels of dexamethasone
    d. high levels of epinephrine

19. In one study, creative writers were found to be more likely to suffer from what disorder than a matched group?
    a. bipolar disorder
    b. anxiety neurosis
    c. schizophrenia
    d. multiple personality

20. Psychoanalytic treatment for depression attempts to have the client
    a. give up the pursuit of a lost object
    b. find an object lost in the past
    c. avoid analysis of present conflicts
    d. control or repress unpleasant feelings

21. Lewinsohn's *Coping with Depression Course* involves all but one of the following. Which of the following activities is not one of Lewinsohn's therapeutic steps?
    a. developing relaxation skills
    b. engaging in fun activities
    c. hypnotic exploration of the unconscious
    d. acquisition of better social skills

22. Cognitive therapy seeks to help clients recognize cognitive distortions. Which of the following statements is an example of a cognitive distortion?

A

   a. "I know I'm going to flunk this course."
   b. "Stop blaming yourself for everyone else's problems."
   c. "Feeling something doesn't make it so."
   d. "Nobody is destined to be a loser."

23. MAO inhibitors

A

   a. block the activity of an enzyme
   b. stimulate release of neurotransmitters
   c. inhibit reuptake sites on postsynaptic membrane
   d. are safer to take than tricyclics

24. Lithium as a treatment of bipolar disorder

D

   a. is extremely safe with few side effects
   b. has clearly understood pharmacological effects
   c. can be discontinued once normal mood is obtained
   d. is more effective in treating manic episodes

25. Electroconvulsive therapy has been found to

C

   a. have less severe side effects than drug therapy
   b. be more effective than drug therapy
   c. be no more effective than simulated ECT in recent studies
   d. be clearly more effective if delivered bilaterally

26. Among which age group are suicide rates the highest?

D

   a. young children
   b. adolescents
   c. mature adults
   d. the elderly

27. Which theory of suicide suggests and emphasizes that people committing suicide do so because they believe that it will solve their problems?

D

   a. Psychoanalytic
   b. Existential-humanist
   c. sociocultural
   d. social-learning

28. If you think you are dealing with a person who is considering committing suicide, what should you say?

C

   a. "You're talking crazy."
   b. "Let's go talk to your folks about it."
   c. "Come with me and we'll find some help."
   d. "You're just being silly."

TERMS AND CONCEPTS

Lesson 1
bereavement (252)
bipolar disorder (257)
cyclothymia (259)
double depression (257)
dysthymia (257)
endogenous depression (254)
hypo-manic episodes (259)
major depression (250)
manic episodes (258)
mood disorders (250)
moods (250)
postpartum depression (256)
rapid flight of ideas (258)
reactive depression (254)
seasonal affective disorder (255)
the bipolar disorders (251)
the depressive disorders (251)

Lesson 2
Aaron Beck (263)
ambivalent (260)
automatic thoughts (267)
catastrophizing (266)
catecholamine hypothesis (271)
cognitive distortions (263)
Cognitive theory (263)
cognitive-specificity hypothesis (267)
Humanist-Existential Theory (261)
Interactional theory (262)
introject (260)
learned helplessness theory (269)
Learning Theory (262)
musterbation (266)
negative view of oneself (263)
negative view of the environment (263)
negative view of the future (263)
Psychodynamic theory (260)
reformulated helplessness theory (270)
selective abstraction (266)
self-focusing model (260)
tricyclics and monamine oxidase inhibitors (273)

Lesson 3
antidepressant drug therapy (277)
behavioral treatment (275)
cognitive therapy (276)
Coping with Depression Course (275)
electroconvulsive therapy (280)
humanist-existential treatment (274)
lithium therapy (280)
Psychodynamic treatment (274)

TYING THINGS TOGETHER

1. Your text examines treatment for mood disorders separately; however, most treatment in the real world is eclectic. Assume that you are confronted with a person who suffers from major depression. Outline a program which would consist of a combination of biological, behavioral, and cognitive treatments. Be as specific about the sequencing and intermixing of treatments as possible.

2. Predicting suicide are preventing suicide are closely related. Identify the factors that predict that a suicide attempt might be imminent in a person of your own age. Explain what you would do to help prevent this suicide. Finally, discuss why all suicides cannot be prevented.

ANSWERS

Lesson 1	Lesson 2		Lesson 3
1 l	1 e	11 q	1 h
2 m	2 u	12 f	2 d
3 g	3 p	13 i	3 f
4 c	4 b	14 d	4 c
5 k	5 m	15 s	5 a
6 j	6 l	16 r	6 e
7 f	7 t	17 v	7 g
8 d	8 n	18 g	8 b
9 n	9 h	19 k	
10 p	10 a	20 c	
11 e		21 j	
12 o		22 o	
13 q			
14 i			
15 a			
16 b			
17 h			

True-False
answers

1	F	11	F
2	F	12	T
3	F	13	F
4	T	14	T
5	T	15	F
6	T	16	F
7	F	17	F
8	F	18	T
9	T	19	F
10	F	20	F
		21	F
		22	F
		23	F
		24	F
		25	F
		26	T
		27	F
		28	F

Multiple-Choice
answers

1	a	11	d
2	a	12	d
3	c	13	c
4	b	14	c
5	c	15	a
6	a	16	a
7	d	17	a
8	a	18	a
9	d	19	a
10	b	20	a
		21	c
		22	a
		23	a
		24	d
		25	c
		26	d
		27	d
		28	c

9 Disorders of Personality and Impulse Control

OVERVIEW

In learning about the classification of abnormal behavior back in Chapter 3, you learned that personality disorders were classified on Axis II of DSM-III-R. This chapter considers those personality disorders. You will learn the defining features of personality disorders--the things they have in common that serve to separate them from other behavior disorders. Personality disorder are divided into three clusters based on types of behavior. You will learn about these three clusters and the specific personality disorders that fall within them. Consideration of personality disorders is not complete without mention of some new personality disorders that are under consideration and a discussion of the problems in classification of personality disorders. Rathus and Nevid cheerfully oblige, providing sections on these topics. Theoretical perspectives and treatment of personality disorders are very brief sections. If you have been progressing through the text chronologically, you should find the section on theoretical perspectives to be straightforward and relatively easy. Personality disorders are viewed as very resistent to change, making treatment a difficult task. In the treatment section the authors of the text give you information to help you develop a real appreciation for the therapists' views of what they are up against.

The chapter also includes a section on impulse control, which we have separated as a lesson in the study guide. If you have ever wondered about wealthy individuals arrested for shoplifting things they could have easily afforded, or if you have been following the demise of Pete Rose, the extraordinary baseball player and manager who literally gambled away his chances at the baseball hall of fame, this section will be of interest to you. The characteristics and treatment of pathological gambling and kleptomania are carefully outlined in the final section of this chapter.

CHAPTER OUTLINE, LESSONS & LEARNING OBJECTIVES

Lesson 1. Introduction to personality disorders. (291-294)
TYPES OF PERSONALITY DISORDERS. (291-292)
1. Define the common features of personality disorders.
2. Describe the different clusters of personality disorders.

PERSONALITY DISORDERS CHARACTERIZED BY ODD OR ECCENTRIC BEHAVIOR. (292-294)

3. Understand the paranoid, schizoid and schizotypal personality disorders.

Lesson 2. Antisocial, borderline, histrionic and narcissistic personality disorders. (294-302)

PERSONALITY DISORDERS CHARACTERIZED BY DRAMATIC EMOTIONAL, OR ERRATIC BEHAVIOR. (294-302)

4. Understand the antisocial, borderline, histrionic and narcissistic personality disorders.

Lesson 3. Personality disorders characterized by anxious or fearful behavior, proposed personality disorders and problems with classification of personality disorders. (302-310)

PERSONALITY DISORDERS CHARACTERIZED BY ANXIOUS OR FEARFUL BEHAVIOR. (302-305)

5. Understand avoidant, dependent and obsessive-compulsive personality disorders.

PROPOSED PERSONALITY DISORDERS "NEEDING FURTHER STUDY." (306)

6. Understand proposed sadistic and self-defeating personality disorders, and their controversies.
7. Describe the reasons why researchers believe that women who remain in abusive relationships should be perceived as trauma survivors, not masochists.

PROBLEMS WITH CLASSIFICATION OF PERSONALITY DISORDERS. (306-310)

8. Describe the controversies in classifying personality disorders.

Lesson 4. Theoretical perspectives and treatment of personality disorders. (310-320)
THEORETICAL PERSPECTIVES. (310-317)

9. Understand theoretical perspectives of personality disorders.

TREATMENT. (317-320)

10. Describe the approaches to treatment of personality disorders and the difficulties faced by therapists in treating people with these disorders.

Lesson 5. Impulse disorders. (320-324)
IMPULSE DISORDERS. (320-324)

11. Describe the common features of impulse disorders.
12. Discuss the features and treatments of pathological gambling.
13. Discuss the features of kleptomania.

Mastering Lesson 1. Introduction to personality disorders. (291-294)

In mastering this lesson you will learn what personality disorders are. That is, the characteristics that set this family of disorders apart from other kinds of abnormal behavior. You will also learn the three clusters of personality disorders in DSM-III-R that form the basis for the organization of much of this chapter. Another three-way association must be learned: The cluster name, its defining behavior and the specific personality disorders that fall within it. The matching section that follows will help you become fluent with these associations as well as some of the basic terminology of personality disorders.

In some ways it is best to jump right in and see some concrete examples when you encounter a classification scheme. We have done this in lesson one, including the first cluster of personality disorders. This will give you some very concrete experience with the overall classification scheme, while you learn about the first cluster. In studying this section, you should mentally "step back to view the bigger picture" of personality disorders at least once or twice. You should be able to recognize, for example, how the schizoid personality disorder got classified into Cluster A and why it is a personality disorder at all.

Match the following terms and concepts with the correct definition or description or explanation.

1. _C_ anxious or fearful
2. _F_ Cluster A PSS
3. _D_ Cluster B ABHN
4. _E_ Cluster C A,D,OC,P-A
5. _J_ ego-dystonic
6. _I_ ego-syntonic
7. _A_ odd or eccentric
8. _B_ overly dramatic, emotional, or erratic
9. _H_ paranoid personality disorder
10. _K_ personality disorder
11. _G_ schizoid personality disorder
12. _L_ schizotypal personality disorder

a. behaviors characteristic of Cluster A
b. behaviors characteristic of Cluster B
c. behaviors characteristic of Cluster C
d. antisocial, borderline, histrionic and narcissistic personality disorders
e. avoidant, dependent obsessive-compulsive and passive-aggressive personality disorders
f. paranoid, schizoid and schizotypal personality disorders
g. social isolate, rarely shows strong emotion
h. unwarranted suspicion, over-sensitivity to criticism, hypervigilant, but absence of delusions
i. perception that behavior and feelings are natural part of self
j. perception that feelings and behavior are foreign to one's self-identity
k. maladaptive and excessively rigid pattern of relating to others
l. eccentric in any of a variety of ways, though not disturbed to the extent of schizophrenia

Mastering Lesson 2. Antisocial, borderline, histrionic and narcissistic personality disorders (294-302).

This lesson covers the personality disorders included in Cluster B. They are characterized by dramatic emotional behavior or by erratic behavior. In mastering this lesson, you should learn the clinical characteristics of each of these disorders as well as understanding why they are grouped in Cluster B. One of the disorders in this group, antisocial personality disorder, has received a great deal of popular attention and is therefore covered in more depth. The shortness of the matching exercise reflects the emphasis on relationships rather than new vocabulary to be learned.

Match the following terms and concepts with the correct definition or description or explanation.

1. C antisocial personality disorder
2. B borderline personality disorder
3. F Cleckley's clinical profile
4. D histrionic personality disorder
5. E narcissistic personality disorder
6. A normal self-interest
7. G perseveration

a. healthy adjustment to insecurity
b. unstable self-image, relationships and moods
c. impulsive, fail to live up to commitments, disregard rights of others and lack anxiety or guilt over doing so
d. excessive need for praise and approval; desire to be center of attention
e. extreme self-infatuation, absorbed in self, lack empathy for others
f. includes superficial charm and intelligence, lack of remorse or shame, inability to experience love or genuine emotion among ten characteristics of antisocial personality
g. a response deficit characterized by insensitivity to punishment

Mastering Lesson 3. Personality disorders characterized by anxious or fearful behavior, proposed personality disorders and problems with classification of personality disorders (302-310).

This is a catch-all lesson to help you learn several short sections in the text. It includes the personality disorders in Cluster C, and some proposed disorders that are somewhat controversial. The controversy about proposed disorders represents a convenient transition to the discussion of controversies with personality disorders more generally.

In mastering this lesson pay particular attention to features that allow you to distinguish the disorders from other disorders that you have already learned about. For example, you should be able to figure out how obsessive-compulsive personality disorder differs from the obsessive-compulsive disorder in the anxiety disorders presented in chapter six. The matching section which begins on the next page will help you with the technical vocabulary, but there is much richness in the cases presented and narrative to be learned beyond the vocabulary.

Match the following terms and concepts with the correct definition or description or explanation.

1. _D_ avoidant personality disorder
2. _C_ blaming victim of abusive relationship
3. _F_ dependent personality disorder
4. _B_ evasion of criminal responsibility by mental defect
5. _H_ obsessive-compulsive personality disorder
6. _I_ passive-aggressive personality disorder
7. _E_ problems with classification of personality disorders
8. _A_ sadistic personality disorder
9. _G_ self-defeating personality disorder

a. proposed disorder characterized by intentional cruelty, lack of empathy for others
b. major concern about adopting sadistic personality disorder
c. major concern about adopting self-defeating personality disorder
d. social isolate who desperately wants social relationships
e. reliability, validity, overlap and inability to distinguish among normal and abnormal behavior variations are the major ones
f. these individuals find doing things on their own to be exceedingly difficult
g. proposed disorder characterized by long-standing patterns of behavior including rejection of help, attraction to others who mistreat them
h. orderly, perfectionistic rigid individual who has no obsessions or compulsions, has problems coping with ambiguity
i. persistent, long-standing expression of hostility by failure to comply with requests; this noncompliance eventually becoming self-defeating

Mastering Lesson 4. Theoretical perspectives and treatment of personality disorders. (310-320)

This lesson begins with theoretical perspectives. The first thing you will notice is that the psychodynamic perspectives (yes, plural) include views of Hans Kohut, Otto Kemberg and Margaret Maher. You will learn to associate these theorists with their views and recognize that all three represent psychodynamic perspectives.

Personality disorders are highly resistent to change. The chapter begins by telling you some of the reasons that this is so. Most of the coverage in this section deals with treatments emerging from the behavioral and cognitive-behavioral perspectives. These treatments have met with limited success (remember, we said these disorders are difficult to treat) that exceeds the efficacy of other forms of treatment.

Match the following terms and concepts with the correct definition or description or explanation.

1. _I_ biological treatment
2. _J_ emotional responsiveness
3. _P_ Family perspectives
4. _G_ genetic factors
5. _L_ Hans Kohut
6. _E_ Margaret Maher
7. _B_ optimal level of arousal
8. _N_ Otto Kemberg
9. _D_ private self-consciousness
10. _A_ psychodynamic therapy
11. _O_ rational-emotive therapy
12. _M_ self-psychology
13. _K_ separation-individuation
14. _Q_ supermales
15. _H_ Theodore Millon
16. _C_ token economy
17. _R_ Ullmann and Krasner
18. _F_ Walter Mischel

a. ineffective with personality disorders
b. antisocial personalities tend to be sensation seekers
c. systematic reinforcement of prosocial behaviors and extinction of antisocial actions
d. careful self-monitoring of one's behavior results in consistency of behavior across situations
e. psychodynamic theorist, views borderline personality disorders as related to childhood separation from mother figure
f. learning theorist, views behavior as situationally specific and personality disorders as behavior disorders
g. determined by study of relatives of persons displaying personality disorders
h. learning theorist, views histrionic personality disorder as result of inconsistent reinforcement by parents
i. drugs may relieve distress of personality disorders but do little to alter long-standing patterns of maladaptive behavior
j. biological view that antisocial personality disorder results from lack of anticipatory anxiety about being apprehended or punished
k. the process of differentiating one's sense of identity from one's mother
l. psychodynamic theorist, related narcissistic personality disorder to lack of parental empathy and support
m. view that an insecure self lies beneath the narcissistic personality disorder
n. psychodynamic theorist, views borderline personality disorder as related to pre-Oedipal failure to develop self-image
o. an effective means of dealing with management of anger problems that often accompany personality disorders
p. the McCords pointed to parental rejection and neglect as the source of antisocial personality
q. chromosomal abnormality characterized by XYY sex-chromosomal pattern, was incorrectly thought to be related to violence
r. learning perspective, proposed that antisocial personality disorders are failure to respond to social reinforcers

Mastering Lesson 5. Impulse disorders. (320-324).

This lesson focuses on the impulse disorders. Begin this lesson by learning the three diagnostic features that all of the impulse disorders share in common. The two specific impulse disorders covered in this text are pathological gambling and kleptomania. We think you will find that both are fascinating enough to maintain your interest. In fact, it is quite likely that you are already familiar with individuals suffering from impulse disorders, either first-hand in someone you personally know or through the news media. Beware! Do not assume that reading newspaper accounts of Pete Rose allows you to master the pathological gambling disorder in this lesson. Your knowledge is at the everyday level. Psychologists focus on certain key features. You must learn the characteristics that psychologists use to classify these impulse disorders. Hidden in the textbook narrative is a bit of theoretical perspective and treatment information. If you are a good student, you will be able to ferret this information out without it having the usual section headings. The mastery section below gets you started with the basic terminology of the lesson.

Match the following terms and concepts with the correct definition or description or explanation.

1. C covert sensitization
2. D desperation phase
3. E impulse control disorders
4. E kleptomania
5. A losing phase
6. H low self-esteem
7. G pathological gambling
8. B winning phase

a. wagering borrowed money to get even
b. nearly half of pathological gamblers experienced a big win here
c. behavioral treatment involving imagined pairing of aversive stimuli with undesired behavior to reduce impulsive behaviors
d. obsession with winning in order to break even unstabilizes personal, family or occupational roles leading to irrational gambling risks
e. compulsive stealing, usually involving items of little value
f. failure to resist impulse, drive or temptation to engage in action harmful to self or others
g. involves repeated failure to resist the urge to gamble resulting in impairment of functioning in personal, family or occupational roles
h. many compulsive gamblers have this and use gambling as a means (usually unsuccessful) of boosting it

PRACTICE EXAMS

<u>Exam 1. (true-false).</u>
Indicate whether each of the following statements is True or False. Question numbers correspond to learning objectives from which the questions were drawn.

1. F Personality disorders include inflexible ways of behaving that do not cause significant impairment of functioning.
2. F Anxious and fearful behavior is characteristic of Cluster A personality disorders.
3. T Paranoid personality disorder EXCLUDES paranoid delusions and magical thinking.
4. F Borderline personality disorder is characterized by aloofness and independence from others.

5. E The obsessive-compulsive personality disorder is characterized by long-standing obsessions and compulsions.
6. T Appeal to the salvation ethic is one type of rationalization commonly used by a victim of spouse abuse for remaining in the relationship.
7. T Strube (1988) showed that battered wives were impaired in their ability to think clearly enough to engage in problem solving.
8. T Personality disorders do not explain the reasons for their characteristic behaviors.
9. E Traditional Freudian theory focused on anal fixation problems as the foundation for personality disorders.
10. T A difficulty for all therapeutic efforts with antisocial personality disorder is the inability to establish trust and rapport.
11. E After an impulsive act is committed the person nearly always experiences guilt or regret.
12. F Pathological gamblers are most likely to seek treatment during the losing phase.
13. T Psychodynamic perspectives have viewed kleptomania as stealing objects that were symbolic of the penis as defenses against penis envy or castration anxiety

Exam 2 (multiple-choice)

Select the single, best answer for each question. Question numbers correspond to learning objectives from which the questions were drawn.

1. Analogy: Personality disorders are to _____ as other disorders are to _____.
   a. axis II; axis IV
   b. ego-systonic; ego-dystonic
   c. ego-dystonic; ego-systonic
   d. odd or eccentric; anxious or fearful

2. Which of the following personality disorders fall into Cluster B?
   a. histrionic, obsessive-compulsive
   b. dependent, passive-aggressive
   c. schizoid, paranoid
   d. antisocial, narcissistic

3. Analogy: Schizotypal is to schizoid as
   a. general eccentric is to social isolate
   b. social isolate is to general eccentric
   c. suspicious is to social isolate
   d. general eccentric is to suspicious

4. Which of these is not part of Cleckley's clinical profile of antisocial personality disorder?
   a. responding to setbacks with depression or fury
   b. lack of remorse or shame
   c. inability to profit from experience
   d. superficial charm and intelligence

5. Analogy: fear of rejection is to lack of interest in social relations as
    a. dependent personality disorder is to schizotypal personality disorder
    b. schizotypal personality disorder is to avoidant personality disorder
    c. avoidant personality disorder is to schizoid personality disorder
    d. schizoid personality disorder is to avoidant personality disorder

6. The controversy over whether to adopt the proposed sadistic personality disorder centers around the
    a. ability to clearly define sadistic behavior
    b. possibility that it will allow individuals to avoid criminal responsibility for their sadistic acts
    c. decision of whether to separate mental cruelty from physical cruelty
    d. ability to also determine the presence of masochism

7. Strube's (1988) research showed that victims of spouse abuse
    a. all suffered from self-defeating personality disorder
    b. tend to blame their spouses for physical injury but not mental duress
    c. were similar to former hostage or kidnap victims who had survived their traumas
    d. rarely seek professional assistance

8. Which of the following is not a major controversy in the classification of personality disorders?
    a. too many cases that fit two or more diagnostic categories
    b. excessive ambiguity in diagnostic criteria
    c. inclusion of traits that are normal in lesser degree as key diagnostic criteria
    d. debate as to whether they need a separate axis in DSM-III-R or should be included in Axis I

9. Research with "supermales", individuals with XYY sex chromosomal anomalies showed that
    a. most violent male offenders were not supermales
    b. most violent male offenders were supermales
    c. supermales tended to be superficially bright and friendly
    d. athletes tended to be supermales

10. Which of the following conclusions can be drawn from research using token economies to reinforce prosocial behavior and extinguish antisocial behavior?
    a. token economies were ineffective in altering antisocial behavior
    b. token economies must be combined with cognitive treatment for anger management
    c. token economies are effective in the treatment of antisocial personality disorders
    d. token economies can reduce antisocial behavior but it is unclear whether they can prevent adolescents from developing antisocial personality disorders as adults

11. Impulse disorders have all of these features in common except
    a. increased arousal prior to committing the impulsive act
    b. experiencing the act as ego-dystonic during the time it is committed
    c. experience of pleasure when committing the impulsive act
    d. failure to resist impulse, drive or temptation to engage in behavior harmful to self or others

12. Pathological gambling is motivated more by _____ than by
_____.
    a. winning; losing
    b. losing; winning
    c. excitement of wagering; pursuit of money
    d. pursuit of money; excitement of wagering

13. Kleptomania
    a. is the most common cause of shoplifting
    b. is motivated primarily by poverty
    c. is more common among women than among men
    d. rarely results in arrest due to experience of the kleptomaniac

TERMS AND CONCEPTS

Lesson 1
Cluster A (292)
Cluster B (292)
Cluster C (292)
ego-dystonic (292)
ego-syntonic (292)
paranoid personality
disorder (292)
personality disorder (292)
schizoid personality
disorder (293)
schizotypal personality
disorder (293)

Lesson 2
antisocial personality
disorder (294)
borderline personality
disorder (298)
Cleckley's clinical profile
(297)
histrionic personality
disorder (299)
narcissistic personality
disorder (300)
normal self-interest (300)
perseveration (297)

Lesson 3
avoidant personality
disorder (302)
dependent personality
disorder (303)
obsessive-compulsive
personality disorder (304)
passive-aggressive
personality disorder (305)
sadistic personality
disorder (306)
self-defeating personality
disorder (306)

Lesson 4
emotional responsiveness
(315)
Family perspectives (313)
genetic factors (314)
Hans Kohut (310)
Margaret Maher (311)
optimal level of arousal
(315)
Otto Kemberg (311)
private self-consciousness
(313)

psychodynamic therapy
(317)
rational-emotive therapy
(319)
self-psychology (310)
separation-individuation
(311)
supermales (314)
Theodore Millon (312)
token economy (318)
Ullmann and Krasner
(312)
Walter Mischel (312)

Lesson 5
covert sensitization (324)
desperation phase (323)
impulse control disorders
(320)
kleptomania (324)
losing phase (323)
pathological gambling
(320)
winning phase (323)

112

TYING THINGS TOGETHER

1. Make a chart showing the relationships of the terminology in this chapter. The best chart might be structured like a corporate organizational chart. Leave room to write in definitions and characteristics and you will create a super study aid.

2. Many normal individuals display some of the characteristics of personality disorders but to a lesser degree. Writers sometimes base fictional characters on such individuals. It is not hard to do. Start by thinking of someone you know who displays some of the characteristics of one of the personality disorders in mild form. Then write a description of a fictional character by simply exaggerating these characteristics out of proportion. Share your description with members of your study group--yes, study groups are a good idea. Can members diagnose your fictional character correctly?

3. The saga of Pete Rose's gambling problems was just coming to a close as we wrote this study guide. Since Pete becomes eligible for membership into the Baseball Hall of Fame in 1992, it is likely that news commentary will continue. Your task is to create a case study of Pete from newspaper and magazine sources. Add your own thoughts as to how well the news accounts correspond to the textbook characteristics and whether you think that Pete Rose really suffered from pathological gambling.

ANSWERS

Lesson 1	Lesson 2	Lesson 4	Lesson 5
1 c	1 c	1 i	1 c
2 f	2 b	2 j	2 d
3 d	3 f	3 p	3 f
4 e	4 d	4 g	4 e
5 j	5 e	5 l	5 a
6 i	6 a	6 e	6 h
7 a	7 g	7 b	7 g
8 b		8 n	8 b
9 h	**Lesson 3**	9 d	
10 k	1 d	10 a	
11 g	2 c	11 o	
12 l	3 f	12 m	
	4 b	13 k	
	5 h	14 q	
	6 i	15 h	
	7 e	16 c	
	8 a	17 r	
	9 g	18 f	

True-False answers	Multiple-Choice answers
1 F	1 b
2 F	2 d
3 T	3 a
4 F	4 a
5 F	5 c
6 T	6 b
7 T	7 c
8 T	8 d
9 F	9 a
10 T	10 d
11 F	11 b
12 F	12 c
13 T	13 c

10 Substance Abuse and Dependence

OVERVIEW

This chapter explains the relationship of the use of psychoactive chemicals (in a word, drugs) and abnormal psychology. It begins by asking the question, "When is using drugs abnormal?" After introducing some basic terms and concepts from psychopharmacology the chapter examines drugs, grouped together by pharmaceutical categories. You will need to learn to associate specific drugs with the category name each belongs to. This will help you learn the effects of these drugs, as categories generally have effects in common (though routes of chemical action of specific drugs within a category may differ). You must learn to discuss (list and briefly describe) the major effects of each of the drugs included in the chapter.

The last two lessons in the chapter deal with theoretical perspectives and treatments. In these sections, more so than the corresponding sections of earlier chapters you will find considerable controversy. Different theoretical perspectives have led to treatment goals and strategies that aren't just different, they are strongly opposed to one another. Like personality disorders in chapter nine, drug abuse is not easily treated. Some of the reasons for the difficulty of treatment are the same, others are specific to the effects of the abused substance. You will learn to identify key characteristics of effective treatments for adolescent substance abuse.

CHAPTER OUTLINE, LESSONS & LEARNING OBJECTIVES

Lesson 1.   Introduction to substance abuse. (329-335)
PSYCHOACTIVE SUBSTANCE ABUSE AND DEPENDENCE. (329-335)
1.   Define substance abuse and substance dependence.
2.   Distinguish between psychological and physiological dependence.
SUBSTANCE ABUSE AND ORGANIC MENTAL DISORDERS. (335)
3.   Describe organic mental disorders that are induced by the use of psychoactive substances.

Lesson 2.   Alcohol, barbiturates and minor tranquilizers, and opiate drugs. (335-343)

ALCOHOL. (335-341)

4.   Describe U.S. drinking patterns and prevalences of alcoholism.
5.   List the risk factors for alcoholism and briefly describe each of them.
6.   Discuss the effects of alcohol.

BARBITURATES (SEDATIVES) AND MINOR TRANQUILIZERS. (341)

7.   Discuss the effects of barbiturates and minor tranquilizers.

OPIATES. (341-343)

8.   Discuss the origins and effects of opiate drugs.

Lesson 3.   Stimulants and psychedelics. (343-352)

STIMULANTS. (343-350)

9.   Discuss the effects of amphetamines.
10.   Discuss the effects of cocaine.
11.   Discuss the effects of nicotine and tobacco smoke.

PSYCHEDELICS. (350-352)

12.   Discuss the effects of LSD.
13.   Discuss the effects of PCP.
14.   Discuss the effects of marijuana.

Lesson 4.   Theoretical perspectives. (352-361)

THEORETICAL PERSPECTIVES. (352-361)

15.   Discuss biological, psychodynamic, learning, cognitive and sociocultural approaches to substance abuse and dependence.
16.   Discuss the disease model of substance abuse and dependence.
17.   Discuss genetic factors in alcoholism.

Lesson 5.   Treatment of substance abuse and dependence. (361-368)

TREATMENT. (361-368)

18.   Discuss chemotherapeutic approaches to treatment of substance abuse and dependence.
19.   Discuss nonprofessional support groups, such as AA, and residential treatment programs.
20.   Discuss psychodynamic and behavioral approaches to treatment.
21.   Discuss the controversies concerning controlled drinking treatment strategies.
22.   Discuss the need for, methods of, and evaluation of relapse-prevention training.
23.   Describe some of the characteristics that are believed to be associated with more successful substance abuse programs for adolescents.

Mastering Lesson 1. Introduction to substance abuse. (329-335)

This lesson introduces the basic terminology of substance abuse. Mastery requires that you learn this and how to draw the line between substance use and abuse. You will also learn the major categories of organic mental disorders that involve substance abuse. Learn the terms and concepts of this lesson well. They form the working vocabulary for the remainder of the chapter. Be careful to note the relations among terms. Find out how substance abuse and substance dependence fit together, how addiction relates to psychological and physiological dependence.

These things will make the key terms and concepts part of your working vocabulary. The matching section that follows provides just a beginning.

Match the following terms and concepts with the correct definition or description or explanation.

1. _N_ abstinence syndrome
2. _J_ addiction
3. _M_ delirium
4. _F_ delirium tremens
E 5. _E_ hallucinations
6. _C_ intoxication
7. _B_ physiological dependence
8. _K_ psychoactive
9. _A_ psychological dependence
10. _H_ substance abuse
11. _G_ substance dependence
12. _I_ tachycardia
13. _L_ tolerance
14. _D_ withdrawal

a. impaired control over use of a drug that is not accompanied by physiological dependence
b. symptoms include development of tolerance, abstinence syndrome or both
c. behavior changes induced by chemical actions of psychoactive substances
d. dramatic reduction in intake of an abused substance; produces symptoms characteristic of the specific substance to which the individual is physiologically dependent
e. seeing or hearing things that are not present
f. involve intense autonomic hyperactivity, mental confusions, extreme restlessness
g. behavior indicating impaired ability to control use of a psychoactive substance
h. continued use of a substance despite knowledge that use is causing the individual to suffer physical, psychological, social or occupational problems
i. abnormally rapid heart rate, a component of the effects of alcohol withdrawal
j. everyday term for habitual use of a drug accompanied by signs of physiological dependence
k. describes chemicals which have a psychological effect
l. with continued use of a substance, higher doses are needed to maintain the same effect
m. mental confusion and disorientation combined with inability to focus attention
n. characteristic symptoms following sudden withdrawal or reduction in use of a substance

Mastering Lesson 2. Alcohol, barbiturates and minor tranquilizers, and opiate drugs. (335-343)

This lesson begins with the most abused drug in the United States, alcohol. Largely because of the extent of alcohol abuse you will need to learn about drinking patterns and prevalences. The barbiturates and minor tranquilizers are considered, and opiate drugs presented. As with all drugs in this chapter, mastery requires that you learn about the nature of each class of drug (where it comes from, how it is used, etc.), examples of specific drugs in the class, the physical and behavioral effects of the drug class, whether it produces physiological or psychological dependence or both, and the characteristic abstinence syndrome (if it has one). In fact, a good way to study this lesson and the one that follows is to make a chart to summarize this information across drugs in this chapter (see the first "Tying Things Together" exercise at the end of this study guide chapter).   Although the matching section is long, you will be able to readily relate it to your previous knowledge about substance abuse.

Match the following terms and concepts with the correct definition or description or explanation.

1. N alcohol
2. J alcohol amnestic disorder
K 3. ~~D~~ alcoholism
U 4. ~~E~~ alcoholism risk factors
O 5. ~~O~~ barbiturate addicts *mostly for insomnia*
6. D barbiturate withdrawal *fatal convulsions*
7. V barbiturates *depressants*
8. S cirrhosis of the liver
9. C decreased sexual arousal
10. ~~A~~ depressant drug found in liquor
11. R endorphins
12. ~~F~~ female alcoholics
13. G fetal alcohol syndrome
14. T gout
15. E heroin
16. B increased sexual arousal
17. P light drinking
18. M male alcoholics
19. ~~H~~ minor tranquilizers
20. I opiates
21. L opium poppy
22. Q pain relief

a. alcohol
b. expected effect of alcohol
c. actual effect of alcohol
d. may produce fatal convulsions
e. drug first developed in 1875 to cure morphine addiction
f. tend to drink large amounts of alcohol daily
g. pattern of retarded development and features estimated to affect at least 40% of children born to mothers who drink during pregnancy
h. include valium and librium, are now known to produce psychological dependence
i. principally morphine, heroin and codeine, produce analgesia
j. alcohol induced vitamin B deficiency produces confusion, disorientation and memory loss
k. has no universally accepted definition
l. codeine and morphine are extracted from it
m. tend to alternate between heavy drinking and abstinence
n. the most abused substance in the United States
o. most are middle-aged individuals initially taking this substance to combat insomnia
p. may elevate HDL cholesterol levels reducing heart disease risk, but current data are inconsistent
q. primary medical use of opiate drugs
r. neurotransmitters chemically similar to opiate drugs are thought to be involved in pleasure and pain experiences
s. chronic alcohol use causes protein deficiency which results in this
t. increased uric acid levels resulting from alcohol metabolism can result in this
u. includes family history, age, sex, social class and race
v. depressant drugs used medically to alleviate anxiety and insomnia

Mastering Lesson 3. Stimulants and psychedelics (343-352)

This lesson continues the consideration of specific drugs, exploring three psychoactive drugs classified as stimulants and three more classified as psychedelics. To master this lesson you must learn how drugs in each category work, which category drugs fall in and their specific effects.

If you are making a matrix (table) to summarize the drugs in this chapter, you should fill in the appropriate parts of your matrix as you encounter key ideas in this lesson. Look at the first exercise in "Tying Things Together" at the end of this study guide chapter.

Match the following terms and concepts with the correct definition or description or explanation.

1. A amotivational syndrome
2. J amphetamine psychosis
3. H amphetamines
4. P cocaine
5. C cocaine health risks
6. D epinephrine release
7. F freebasing
8. L hashish
9. E LSD
10. I marijuana
11. K nicotine
12. G norepinephrine and dopamine
13. B PCP
14. O psychedelics
15. N stimulants
16. M THC

a. low achievement motivation ambition and ability to concentrate correlated with regular marijuana use in college students

b. "angel dust", produces dissociation between self and environment

c. heart irregularities, seizures, increased blood pressure and body temperature

d. produced by nicotine, generates burst of autonomic activity

e. produces visual hallucinations by decreasing serotonin action and increasing dopamine activity

f. heating cocaine powder with ether to release its psychoactive chemical base which is then inhaled

g. neurotransmitters whose release is expedited and/or reuptake inhibited by stimulant drugs

h. stimulants initially used to extend vigilance, common abuse pattern is extended high followed by "crash" to period of deep sleep and/or depression

i. the nation's most popular illicit drug, produces mild hallucinations

j. drug-induced state that mimics paranoid schizophrenia

k. stimulant drug that only rarely produces intoxication but does produce tolerance and abstinence syndromes

l. psychoactive substance derived from resin of marijuana plant

m. most highly concentrated in resins of female marijuana plant

n. class of psychoactive substances that increase nervous system activity

o. class of psychoactive substances that produce sensory distortions or hallucinations, primarily of color perception and hearing

p. natural stimulant extracted from the cocoa plant

Mastering Lesson 4. Theoretical perspectives. (352-361)

The theoretical perspectives on substance abuse have generated considerable research, particularly with alcohol abuse (because of its prevalence in our society). The insights and theories that have resulted from this research are perhaps better associated with the model from which they come rather than with a specific drug class other than alcohol. This simplifies the learning needed to master this lesson. The matching section below provides some fluency-building practice with basic terms and concepts.

Match the following terms and concepts with the correct definition or description or explanation.

1. _C_ biological perspectives
2. _L_ classical conditioning perspective
3. _A_ cognitive perspective
4. _E_ disease model
5. _D_ genetics of alcohol abuse
6. _I_ observational learning perspective
7. _M_ one drink-one drunk
8. _B_ operant conditioning perspective
9. _F_ outcome expectancies
10. _K_ psychodynamic perspective
11. _H_ self-awareness model
12. _J_ self-efficacy expectations
13. _G_ sociocultural perspective

a. expectancies more important than physiological effects
b. focus on reinforcing effects of drugs
c. biology of abstinence syndromes, genetic factors and disease model represent the three major contributions.
d. biological sons of alcoholic parents are at risk
e. assumes that alcoholism is an irreversible disease state
f. people who expect positive outcomes from drug use more likely to become abusers
g. best predictor of adolescent drug use is use by friends
h. high self-awareness people experiencing failure are most likely to abuse alcohol
i. modeling influences heavy social drinkers, but not light drinkers
j. alcohol and cocaine form the focus of this theory
k. alcoholism and smoking are signs of oral fixations
l. craving viewed not as drug effect per se, but as conditioned response associated with circumstances of drug use
m. an expectancy taught in AA; cognitive psychologists believe that the expectancy creates a self-fulfilling prophesy

Mastering Lesson 5. Treatment of substance abuse and dependence. (361-368)

Rathus and Nevid begin this section by pointing out that treatment of substance abuse is very frustrating. It is easy to get clients through abstinence syndromes, but a far different matter to enable them to discontinue their abuse in the long term. This is true in spite of the variety of treatments available from professional and nonprofessional sources. Keep this thought in mind as you learn about specific treatments: The value of a treatment for substance abuse depends mostly upon the likelihood that clients will be able to avoid returning to abuse and dependence of the substance after treatment. The matching section that follows should help you with the basic terminology for this lesson.

Match the following terms and concepts with the correct definition or description or explanation.

1. _E_ abstinence violation effect
2. _G_ Al-Anon
3. _L_ antidepressants
4. _D_ aversive conditioning
5. _O_ behavioral approaches
6. _Q_ covert sensitization
7. _N_ detoxification
8. _K_ disulfiram
9. _B_ methadone maintenance
10. _F_ naloxone
11. _I_ nicotine chewing gum
12. _M_ psychodynamic approaches
13. _H_ relapse-prevention training
14. _C_ residential approaches
15. _A_ self-control strategies
16. _J_ self-help groups
17. _P_ skills training

a. a grouping of therapies which focus on the ABCs of substance abuse, helping clients alter antecedents, behaviors and consequences involved in substance abuse

b. a slow-acting opiate used in treatment of heroin addiction

c. extended detoxification and therapy in hospitals or therapeutic communities are helpful for clients lacking self-control and those who cannot tolerate withdrawal symptoms

d. treatments based on pairing of noxious stimuli with drug abuse of drug abuse stimuli

e. tendency to over-react to a single instance of drug use and "give up" returning to substance abuse

f. a drug which blocks the action of opiate drugs used to discourage return to opiate abuse

g. a spin-off of AA designed to provide support for families of alcoholics

h. teaching clients how to prevent lapses from resulting in a return to substance dependence

i. a review of placebo-control studies supports its use in combination with behavior therapy to help people stop smoking

j. promote complete abstinence as the treatment goal, rely on social support to help clients remain abstinent

k. when combined with alcohol produces a strong aversion reaction; is used to discourage use of alcohol

l. early results show these drugs may help prevent relapse in cocaine abuse

m. evidence supporting their efficacy is limited to case studies

n. helping a physiologically dependent individual through the abstinence syndrome

o. views substance abuse as a behavior problem rather than a disease state

p. treatments based on teaching better interpersonal relations skill to provide an adaptive alternative to drug use

q. treatments based on imagined pairing of noxious stimuli with drug abuse of drug abuse stimuli

PRACTICE EXAMS

<u>Exam 1. (true-false).</u>
Indicate whether each of the following statements is **True** or **False**. Question numbers correspond to learning objectives from which the questions were drawn.

1. _F_ A duration of at least six months is required for diagnosis of substance abuse in DSM-III-R.
2. _F_ Tolerance is characteristic of both physiological and psychological dependence.
3. _T_ Intoxication is also referred to as drunkenness or being high.
4. _F_ Cocaine is the most widely abused substance in the United States.
5. _T_ The best predictor of alcohol abuse is a family history of this disorder.
6. _F_ Research has shown that the aggression-increasing effect of alcohol is due to people's stereotypic expectations rather than to physiologically mediated effects.
7. _F_ Minor tranquilizers, including valium and librium reduce anxiety without producing sedation.
8. _T_ Users claim that heroin produces sufficient sedation to eliminate interest in the major human sources of pleasure.
9. _F_ Suicide among amphetamine abusers rarely occurs, and when it does attempts are made during the extended high period of abuse.
10. _T_ Cocaine not only enhances performance, but also builds confidence; these properties have popularized it among professional athletes.
11. _T_ Smokers are likely to smoke more during stress because stress increases the rate of nicotine release.
12. _T_ LSD users who experience flashbacks tend to be more oriented towards fantasy and prone to focusing on internal sensory information.
13. _F_ PCP was originally developed as a designer drug to avoid prosecution for distribution of illegal substances.
14. _F_ Hashish is a potent form of marijuana derived from distillation of THC from plant leaves.
15. _F_ According to the cognitive view, the belief that one sip of alcohol will cause a binge is more likely the cause of the binge than the biological effects of the alcohol itself.
16. _F_ Modern professionals are in general agreement that the disease model accurately describes substance abuse.
17. _T_ The best conclusion that can be drawn from genetic research on alcoholism is that genetic factors outweigh environmental factors for men while environmental factors dominate in women.
18. _T_ Taking naloxone prevents subsequent use of opiate drugs from producing any effect.
19. _T_ Residential treatment programs suffer from high initial drop-out rates which make it difficult to assess their effectiveness.
20. _F_ The large number of successful case studies of psychodynamic treatment of substance abuse clearly demonstrate its effectiveness.
21. _F_ Controlled-drinking treatment strategies will not work with "true" alcoholics.
22. _T_ Relapse prevention training is important because of the very poor long-term fillip results from substance abuse treatments.
23. _F_ Therapists who were most successful in working with adolescents were themselves under 23 years of age.

122

Select the single, best answer for each question. Question numbers correspond to learning objectives from which the questions were drawn.

1. All of the following are instances of substance abuse <u>except</u>
   a. repeatedly driving while intoxicated
   b. losing sales due to using cocaine prior to sales presentation with six major clients this month
   c. missing work 13 days in the last six weeks due to alcohol use
   d. smoking marijuana at a friend's house on Saturday nights for the last year

2. Which of the following is not a diagnostic criteria for psychoactive substance dependence?
   a. inability to reduce drug use
   b. experiencing intoxication with smaller amounts of the psychoactive substance
   c. spending increased time obtaining, using and recovering from substance use
   d. use of the substance to prevent withdrawal symptoms

3. Psychoactive substances can produce organic mental disorders by producing effects on the brain
   a. seen only as intoxication
   b. seen only as abstinence syndromes
   c. seen as either abstinence syndrome or intoxication
   d. must be seen as both a and b together

4. Which of the following is <u>not</u> one of the principle patterns of chronic alcohol abuse?
   a. heavy consumption of alcohol when alone at home
   b. periods of binge drinking separated by long periods of abstinence
   c. regular consumption of large quantities of alcohol
   d. heavy weekend drinking

5. Risk factors for alcoholism include
   a. sex, age, social class, race and antisocial personality disorder
   b. age, social class, alcoholism in family, mood disorders, obsessive-compulsive personality disorder
   c. alcoholism in family, race, depression, tobacco use
   d. tobacco use, borderline personality disorder, race, social class, sex

6. Fetal alcohol syndrome
   a. requires the mother to drink during the third trimester of pregnancy
   b. includes symptoms of narrowly spaced eyes, flattened nose and mental retardation
   c. affects all children born to mothers who drank heavily during pregnancy
   d. can occur when the mother drinks only one or two ounces of alcohol per day

7. Barbiturates

C

    a. produce only physiological dependence
    b. produce only psychological dependence
    c. quickly produce both physiological and psychological dependence
    d. produce neither physiological nor psychological dependence

8. The incidence of heroin abuse

B

    a. has declined due to the risk of AIDS from the use of unsterile needles
    b. has remained constant at 1975 levels, probably due to the popularity of cocaine and crack cocaine
    c. is largely confined to younger individuals
    d. among new users occurs primarily in Blacks

9. Amphetamines

C

    a. produce amphetamine psychosis in moderate doses
    b. do not produce tolerance
    c. quickly produce psychological dependence in those who take them to relieve depression
    d. produce neither physiological nor psychological dependence

10. Repeated high-dosage cocaine use

B

    a. is nearly always fatal
    b. can result in anxiety and depression
    c. raises threshold of grand-mal seizures
    d. produces a reverse-tolerance effect

11. Tobacco smoke contains nicotine and

D

    a. chlorinated hydrocarbons
    b. THC
    c. epinephrine
    d. carbon monoxide

12. The psychedelic which produces visual hallucinations by decreasing the action of serotonin is

A

    a. LSD
    b. PCP
    c. THC
    d. marijuana, but only as hashish

13. The psychedelic drug most likely to induce violent or aggressive behavior is

B

    a. LSD
    b. PCP
    c. THC
    d. marijuana, but only as hashish

14. Individuals intoxicated by THC
    a. perceive time as passing more slowly
    b. experience decreased awareness of internal stimuli but increased awareness of external cues
    c. experience decreased awareness of both internal stimuli and external cues
    d. perceive time as passing more rapidly

15. Biological approaches to substance abuse
    a. are inconsistent with the AA approach to treatment of alcoholism
    b. focus on genetic factors, abstinence syndromes and the disease model
    c. have resulted in development of a clear understanding of the biology of cocaine withdrawal
    d. have not been able to differentiate brain wave patterns of biological sons of alcoholics from sons of nonalcoholics

16. The disease model of alcoholism
    a. is consistent with the DSM-III-R classification system
    b. allows for treatment leading to a total cure for alcoholism
    c. is not consistent with genetic information about the causes of alcoholism
    d. leads to conceptualizing excessive drinking as a moral defect

17. Evidence for a genetic basis of alcohol abuse is provided by
    a. adoption studies showing biological sons of alcoholics raised by their biological parents were more likely to become alcoholic than if they were raised by foster parents
    b. evidence that biological children of alcoholics show less relaxation to alcohol increasing the amount they must consume to relax
    c. insignificant differences between MZ and DZ twins in concordance rates
    d. studies which bred rats who were prone to alcohol abuse

18. In order to be effective in helping people stop smoking, nicotine chewing gum
    a. must become a permanent substitute for tobacco
    b. must be combined with other forms of treatment
    c. must be prescribed by a physician
    d. should be used only when the client's craving for a cigarette is low

19. High success rates claimed by AA have been criticized on all of the following grounds except
    a. measures of success limited to self-report
    b. up to 90% of individuals drop out of AA after a few meetings and are not counted in determining success rates
    c. failure to include success rates of control groups
    d. failure to protect anonymity of clients in statistical studies of success

20. Which of the following is not a behavioral treatment for substance abuse?
    a. self-control strategies
    b. aversive conditioning
    c. abstinence violation training
    d. skills training

125

21. Controlled drinking strategies
    a. work best with individuals who can abstain from alcohol
    b. help only those with patterns of heavy binge drinking
    c. are most likely helpful for individuals who have gone through withdrawal symptoms during detoxification
    d. may be effective with younger drinkers, and for those rejecting total abstinence

22. A cognitive-behavior therapy that helps individuals deal with high-risk (for drug use) situations and deal with isolated occasions of drug use without going off the deep end is called
    a. systematic desensitization
    b. coping skills training
    c. relapse prevention training
    d. covert sensitization

23. The most successful substance abuse programs for adolescents included all of these except
    a. special schools for school dropouts
    b. nonconfrontational therapy
    c. vocational counseling
    d. a variety of treatment approaches

TERMS AND CONCEPTS

Lesson 1
abstinence syndrome (332)
addiction (334)
delirium (335)
delirium tremens (335)
hallucinations (335)
intoxication (335)
physiological dependence (333)
psychoactive (330)
psychological dependence (333)
substance abuse (331)
substance dependence (332)
tachycardia (335)
tolerance (332)
withdrawal (332)

Lesson 2
alcohol (335)
alcohol amnestic disorder (338)
alcoholism (336)
alcoholism risk factors (336)
barbiturate withdrawal (341)
barbiturates (341)
cirrhosis of the liver (338)
endorphins (341)
female alcoholics (336)
fetal alcohol syndrome (339)
heroin (342)
male alcoholics (336)

minor tranquilizers (341)
opiates (341)
opium poppy (341)

Lesson 3
amotivational syndrome (352)
amphetamine psychosis (343)
amphetamines (343)
cocaine (343)
cocaine health risks (345)
freebasing (345)
hashish (351)
LSD (350)
marijuana (351)
nicotine (346)
PCP (351)
psychedelics (350)
stimulants (343)
THC (351)

Lesson 4
biological perspectives (353)
classical conditioning perspective (357)
cognitive perspective (359)
disease model (353)
genetics of alcohol abuse (353)
observational learning perspective (357)
one drink-one drunk (353)
operant conditioning perspective (356)

outcome expectancies (358)
psychodynamic perspective (361)
self-awareness model (360)
self-efficacy expectations (359)
sociocultural perspective (360)

Lesson 5
abstinence violation effect (367)
Al-Anon (364)
antidepressants (362)
aversive conditioning (366)
behavioral approaches (365)
covert sensitization (366)
detoxification (362)
disulfiram (362)
methadone maintenance (363)
naloxone (363)
nicotine chewing gum (362)
psychodynamic approaches (365)
relapse-prevention training (366)
residential approaches (364)
self-control strategies (365)
self-help groups (363)
skills training (366)

127

TYING THINGS TOGETHER

1. Keeping track of drug classes, the specific drugs within each class, the physical and psychological effects of these drugs, whether they produce each type of dependence can be a bit of a challenge. A nifty way to study is to make a table somewhat like the one you may have constructed in chapter 6. Get a large sheet of paper or poster board and divide it into 8 columns. Label them "DRUG", "NATURE OF DRUG", "PHYSIOLOGICAL EFFECTS", "PSYCHOLOGICAL EFFECTS", "TOLERANCE", "ABSTINENCE SYNDROME", "DEPENDENCE", "OTHER NOTES". Each time you encounter a drug class, start a new row. Beneath the name of the drug class write some example drugs (ALCOHOL: beer, wine, whiskey). Then fill in the chart as you encounter the key information for that drug class.

ANSWERS

Lesson 1
1 n
2 j
3 m
4 f
5 e
6 c
7 b
8 k
9 a
10 h
11 g
12 i
13 l
14 d

Lesson 2
1 n
2 j
3 k
4 u
5 o
6 d

True-False answers
1 F
2 F
3 T
4 F
5 T
6 T
7 T
8 F
9 F
10 T
11 T
12 T
13 F
14 F
15 T
16 F
17 T
18 T
19 T
20 F
21 F
22 T
23 F

7 v
8 s
9 c
10 a
11 r
12 f
13 g
14 t
15 e
16 b
17 p
18 m
19 h
20 i
21 l
22 q

Lesson 3
1 a
2 j
3 h
4 p
5 c

6 d
7 f
8 l
9 e
10 i
11 k
12 g
13 b
14 o
15 n
16 m

Lesson 4
1 c
2 l
3 a
4 e
5 d
6 i
7 m
8 b
9 f
10 k

Multiple-Choice answers
1 d
2 b
3 c
4 a
5 a
6 d
7 c
8 b
9 c
10 b
11 d
12 a
13 b
14 a
15 c
16 a
17 d
18 b
19 d
20 c
21 d
22 c
23 b

11 h
12 j
13 g

Lesson 5
1 e
2 g
3 l
4 d
5 o
6 q
7 n
8 k
9 b
10 f
11 i
12 m
13 h
14 c
15 a
16 j
17 p

11 Sexual Disorders and Variations in Sexual Behavior

OVERVIEW

In order to understand abnormal sexual behavior, one must first consider what is normal. Rathus and Nevid oblige by discussing cultural differences in what sexual behaviors are considered normal and abnormal, and how American culture has changed its views on sexual behavior since the second world war. With this perspective, the authors then go on to consider a series of sexual disorders. You will notice that the viewpoint of the professional psychologist on sexual disorders (that is presented in the chapter) differs from the everyday view--the viewpoint that you probably hold. Homosexuality, for example, is not itself considered a disorder; problems in adjustment to one's homosexual orientation and the way that orientation is viewed in society can be diagnosed as a sexual disorder. Thus, one of the tricks in learning this chapter is to keep in mind that you are learning the professional psychologist's viewpoint. This will include information such as the diagnostic features of a disorder, its incidence, theoretical perspectives and the efficacy of various treatment methods. Organize your thinking this way and you should find this chapter to be very interesting and not exceedingly difficult.

You should immediately discover that the presentation in this chapter is organized differently than the previous few chapters have been. Rather than considering theoretical perspectives and treatments for all of the disorders of the chapter at the end, this chapter brings up the issues of theory and treatment for each of the relevant disorders as they occur. Anticipating this chapter organization should make learning easier for you.

CHAPTER OUTLINE, LESSONS & LEARNING OBJECTIVES

Lesson 1. American sexual behavior and homosexuality. (373-381)
NORMAL AND ABNORMAL IN AMERICAN SEXUAL BEHAVIOR. (373-377)
1. Describe cultural differences in conceptions of what sexual behaviors are normal and abnormal.
2. Describe the changes that have occurred in American sexual behavior since World War II.

HOMOSEXUALITY. (377-381)
3. Define homosexuality and bisexuality
4. Discuss the psychological adjustment of homosexuals.
5. Discuss theoretical perspectives on homosexuality.
6. Discuss issues concerning "therapy" of homosexuals.

Lesson 2. Gender identity disorders, pornography and rape. (381-390)
GENDER IDENTITY DISORDERS. (381-384)
7. Describe gender identity disorders of childhood and transsexualism.
8. Describe the process of sex reassignment and research results concerning its success rate.
9. Discuss theoretical perspectives on transsexualism.

PORNOGRAPHY. (384-385)
10. Discuss the effects of pornography on sexual arousal and behavior.
11. Discuss the relationship between exposure to violent pornography and aggression against women.

RAPE. (385-390)
12. Describe the incidence of rape.
13. Discuss types of rapists.
14. Discuss theoretical perspectives on the causes of rape.
15. Discuss treatment of rape victims and of rapists.
16. Describe methods of rape prevention.

Lesson 3. Paraphilias. (390-398)
PARAPHILIAS. (390-398)
17. Define and describe the features of various paraphilias
18. Discuss theoretical perspectives on the paraphilias.
19. Describe the effects of childhood sexual abuse on victims.
20. Discuss treatment of persons with paraphilias.

Lesson 4. Sexual dysfunction. (398-410)
SEXUAL DYSFUNCTION. (398-410)
21. Describe the phases of the sexual response cycle.
22. Define and describe the features of various sexual dysfunctions (disorders of desire, arousal, and orgasm).
23. Define and describe the features of sexual disorders involving painful sexual contact.
24. Discuss theoretical perspectives on sexual dysfunctions.
25. Discuss treatment of the sexual dysfunctions.

Mastering Lesson 1. American sexual behavior and homosexuality. (373-381)

In this lesson you will come to appreciate the extent to which one's culture determines what sexual behaviors are normal and abnormal. Many students who take this course are too young to realize just how much the sexual views of American culture have changed. Those of us who are older and perhaps still holding onto values we learned as children may be equally surprised.

This lesson also includes homosexuality. Combining it with the American cultural view does not suggest that homosexuality is accepted by American culture though it is rejected less now than a decade ago. Rather, it is included to even up the length of the lessons in this chapter and to provide the matching exercise that follows in sufficient length to be worthwhile. Learn the professional view of homosexuality, how it implies far more than sexual behavior, the various theoretical perspectives and how treatment has changed in recent years.

Match the following terms and concepts with the correct definition or description or explanation.

1. _C_ biological perspective of homosexuality
2. _A_ bisexuals
3. _I_ ego-dystonic homosexual
4. _M_ homosexuality
5. _H_ Kinsey
6. _D_ learning perspective of homosexuality
7. _K_ marital sex
8. _B_ Masters & Johnson
9. _J_ masturbation
10. _G_ polymorphouslyperverse
11. _F_ premarital intercourse
12. _L_ psychodynamic perspective of homosexuality
13. _E_ treatment of homosexuality

a. respond sexually to both males and females
b. published research on sexual normality in the 1960s that fed the fires of the sexual revolution of the 1960s and 1970s
c. current interest is in prenatal hormonal factors and possible role of genetics
d. classical conditioning results in arousal by stimuli associated with past sexual pleasures
e. conditioning therapies to change sexual orientation and increasingly therapies to help clients adjust to their homosexuality
f. by 1974 more than 95 percent of men and 81 percent of women (age 18-24) had engaged in this behavior
g. Freudian view that young children who have not internalized social inhibitions are open to all forms of sexual stimulation
h. zoologist who published the first scientific surveys of American sexual behavior in the late 1940s and early 1950s
i. refers to homosexuals who reject their sexual orientation; replaced broader category of homosexuality as a sexual disorder
j. now considered normal in spite of continued religious condemnation and notions that it is linked to various physical maladies
k. has increased in diversity of its practice since the Kinsey report
l. mostly relate homosexuality to fixations occurring in the phallic stage
m. a sexual orientation which includes erotic response to members of one's own sex

133

Mastering Lesson 2. Gender identity disorders, pornography and rape. (381-390)

This lesson combines three brief sections of chapter 11. Gender identity disorders refer to a family of disorders in which an individual's biological gender is at odds with a personal (psychological) sense of being male or being female. You must learn about gender disorders of childhood and transsexualism as two major gender identity disorders.

Recent interest on the effects of pornography are probably responsible for its inclusion as a major section in the text. Here you must learn what evidence we have about the various effects claimed for pornography. Clearly this will remain a hotly debated topic from moral and constitutional perspectives. It is important to separate rumor from research evidence in the various psychological effects claimed for pornography.

Like pornography, rape is not a mental disorder (at least not in DSM-III-R). Rape is a criminal activity, but has profound psychological effects on the victim that it is included. This should tell you what to focus on as you master this portion of the lesson. Much of this segment of the lesson focuses on understanding rape trauma syndrome. This focus is also felt in the treatment of rapists, which seems to focus on prevention of additional rape attempts (i.e., protecting us from the rapist). This is in sharp contrast to therapies in earlier chapters that clearly focus on helping the individual who displays the abnormal behavior. The matching section below will help you become familiar and fluent with the diverse ideas in this lesson.

Match the following terms and concepts with the correct definition or description or explanation.

1. F forcible rape
2. H gender identity
3. D gender identity disorder of childhood
4. B gender identity disorder
5. C kinds of (forcible) rape
6. I pornography
7. G rape trauma syndrome
8. A sex reassignment
9. K statutory rape
10. E transsexualism
11. J violent pornography

a. process beginning with assessment of commitment, includes hormone treatments and surgical procedures
b. conflict between biological gender and gender identity
c. categorized by motives as anger, power and sadism
d. less common in boys than girls
e. persistent feelings of being trapped inside body with the wrong (biological) sex
f. use of violence or threat to coerce an individual into sexual intercourse
g. acute period of disorientation, anger, fear, guilt, self-blame followed by a long-term rationalization phase where anxiety, anger, embarrassment fear and guilt diminish with time
h. psychological sense of being male or female
i. produces sexual arousal in both men and women
j. research suggests it may increase male aggression against women
k. intercourse with an individual who has not reached the age of consent

134

Mastering Lesson 3. Paraphilias. (390-398)

Paraphilias all involve sexual arousal to unusual or bizarre objects. Specific paraphilias are named for the object that serves as the arousing stimulus. This should provide a major clue about how to organize your study of this chapter. All of the paraphilias require that the sexual urges, arousal and fantasy be of at least six months duration, and that the individual has either acted on these urges or is significantly distressed by them. Paraphilias other than masochism are extremely rare in females.

The matching section below will enable you to begin building fluency with the major terms. There is a richness in the descriptions of the paraphilias that goes far beyond the basic definitions. Of course this information is so interesting that you will learn it anyway.

Match the following terms and concepts with the correct definition or description or explanation.

1. __K__ exhibitionism
2. __C__ fetishism
3. __I__ frotteurism
4. __J__ incest
5. __L__ paraphilias
6. __A__ partialists
7. __B__ pedophilia
8. __H__ sadomasochism
9. __D__ sexual masochism
10. __G__ sexual sadism
11. __E__ transvestic fetishism
12. __F__ voyeurism

a. an individual with a fetish for a body part such as a foot (preferring the part to the individual)

b. recurrent urges and fantasies regarding sexual activity with prepubescent children

c. sexual arousal to inanimate objects such as clothing

d. sexual urges and arousal focused on being humiliated or made to physically suffer

e. sexual urges and related fantasies involving cross-dressing

f. watching unsuspecting people who are undressed, disrobing or engaging in sexual activity in order to attain sexual excitement

g. sexual urges and arousal focused on making a victim suffer humiliation or physical pain

h. mutually gratifying interaction between a sexual masochist and sexual sadist

i. sexual urges, arousal and fantasy centered on rubbing against or touching a nonconsenting person

j. not a diagnostic category, refers to sexual intercourse among close relatives

k. exposing ones genitals to an unsuspecting stranger in order to surprise shock or sexually arouse the victim

l. sexual arousal to stimuli that are unusual or bizarre

Mastering Lesson 4. Sexual dysfunction. (398-410)

In order to understand sexual dysfunctions it is first necessary to learn about normal sexual function (from a bit more scientific perspective than one's personal experience). You must learn the sequence of phases in the sexual response cycle and what each phase consists of in men and in women. Sexual dysfunctions are divided into four categories in DSM-III-R. You must learn what the categories are, and how sexual behavior in each is dysfunctional (how it differs from the normal sexual response cycle). Finally you must learn some of the major theoretical perspectives about sexual dysfunction and critically examine evidence about the effectiveness of various treatments for the sexual dysfunctions. The matching section that follows will give you some practice that should form a good beginning of familiarity with the information in this lesson.

Match the following terms and concepts with the correct definition or description or explanation.

1. N appetitive phase
2. M dyspareunia
3. H excitement phase
4. F orgasm disorders
5. B orgasm phase
6. A performance anxiety
7. K premature ejaculation
8. J resolution phase
9. E sensate focus exercises
10. L sexual arousal disorders
11. D sexual desire disorders
12. C sexual pain disorders
13. G sexual response cycle
14. I vaginismus

a. fear over ability to perform successfully
b. peak and release of sexual tension
c. dyspareunia and vaginismus
d. the most common presenting problems seen by sex therapists; sexual aversion and hypoactive sexual desire disorder are its types
e. Masters and Johnson's therapeutic technique to counter performance anxiety
f. a trio of disorders: premature ejaculation, inhibited female orgasm and inhibited male orgasm
g. based on research by Masters and Johnson, it consists of appetitive, excitement, orgasm and resolution phases
h. involves erection in men and vaginal lubrication in women
i. involuntary spasm of muscles surrounding vagina making intercourse painful or impossible
j. sense of relaxation, well being and muscle relaxation
k. disorder affecting 30% of the male population at one time or another, more prevalent among younger men
l. disorder of the excitement stage is reserved for persistent problems of erection in men and vaginal lubrication in women
m. pain in genital region associated with sexual intercourse
n. presence of sexual fantasies and desire to engage in sexual activity

PRACTICE EXAMS

Exam 1. (true-false).
Indicate whether each of the following statements is **True** or **False**. Question numbers correspond to learning objectives from which the questions were drawn.

1. T The Mangaian culture is best described as sexually permissive.
2. F Sexual practices in America have become more permissive and this change shows no signs of slowing down.
3. T The desire to form same-sex romantic relationships is a central part of homosexuality.
4. T In spite of discrimination and prejudice, studies of adjustment among homosexual and heterosexual groups found homosexuals to be as well adjusted as their heterosexual counterparts.
5. F Controlled research by learning theorists shows that early punitive relationships with females combined with reinforcement of sexual satisfaction with males can result in a homosexual orientation for men.
6. T In aversive conditioning to change sexual orientation, homosexuals receive electric shocked in the presence of slides depicting homosexual behavior.
7. F A severe case of "tomboyishness" is considered a gender disorder of childhood.
8. T The sex reassignment process begins with determining the competence of the patient to seek reassignment.
9. F Learning theorists point to modeling of homosexual behavior of parents as a causal factor in transsexualism.
10. F In general, viewing pornography results in increases in deviant sexual behavior.
11. T Aggressive pornography may increase rape attempts in men by legitimizing violence against women.
12. T A recent survey of college women reported that over 27% of women had been victims of rape or attempted rape.
13. F Our legal system distinguished statutory rape and sadistic rape as two major forms of illegal forcible sex.
14. T Cognitive psychologists argue that some date rape results from misinterpretation of women's expressed wishes.
15. F Treatment goals for rapists include displacing hostility away from women.
16. F A woman who is attacked should shout "rape" as loudly as she can.
17. F Overt paraphilic behavior is required for diagnosis in DSM-III-R.
18. T Psychodynamic theorists view paraphilias as defenses against castration anxiety.
19. T Abused boys were more likely to be socially isolated and show self-destructive behaviors.
20. T The goal of psychodynamic treatment of paraphilias is to bring sexual conflicts into consciousness where they can be resolved.
21. F During the resolution phase men and women are incapable of reaching orgasm.
22. F Women who require manual clitoral stimulation to reach orgasm during coitus are said to suffer from inhibited female orgasm.
23. F Dyspareunia is a sexual pain disorder affecting only males while vaginismus affects only females.
24. T The behavioral approach emphasizes the role of conditioned anxiety to explain sexual dysfunctions.
25. F Most contemporary sex therapists assume that underlying problems must be identified and brought to a conscious level before sexual dysfunctions can be resolved.

137

Exam 2 (multiple-choice)

Select the single, best answer for each question. Question numbers correspond to learning objectives from which the questions were drawn.

1. Sexual behaviors are considered disorders because
    a. they are harmful to others
    b. they are statistically uncommon in the individual's culture
    c. the individual experiences personal distress associated with the behavior
    d. all of the above can be reasons.

2. Since 1950, the incidence of premarital intercourse in America
    a. reflects a double standard for men and women today more than thirty years ago
    b. increased dramatically in young women to a peak in the 1970s
    c. increased dramatically in young men to a peak in the 1970s and has declined slightly in the 1980s due to AIDS risk
    d. has remained unchanged for both individuals under the age of 25

3. An individual who experiences sexual arousal to members of the same sex
    a. are diagnosed ego dystonic homosexual
    b. are diagnosed bisexual
    c. are diagnosed ego dystonic homosexual only if they reject their sexual orientation
    d. do not suffer from a sexual disorder in American culture

4. Research by Adelman (1977) comparing professionally employed lesbians to heterosexuals found that
    a. heterosexuals were better adjusted
    b. lesbians were better adjusted
    c. though lesbians were more socially isolated the groups were equally well adjusted
    d. both groups had serious adjustment problems to competing in male-dominated professions

5. Research by Bieber claimed that male homosexuality resulted from a combination of a close relationship with a dominant, smothering mother and an empty relationship with a passive father. This research has been highly criticized because
    a. the subjects were all in psychoanalysis but Bieber generalized his findings to include well-adjusted gay men
    b. many heterosexual men are raised in this parental combination
    c. contrary to psychoanalytic theory, many gay males report being closer to their fathers than to their mothers
    d. all of the above are criticisms of Bieber's research

6. Some therapists refuse to try to reverse homosexual orientation
    a. preferring instead to help the individual adjust to his or her sexual orientation
    b. because the success rate for such treatment is very low
    c. due to the risk of AIDS from associating with high risk groups
    d. out of fear that they too will be suspected of being homosexual

7. Which of the following is not a part of the DSM-III-R diagnosis of transsexualism?
   a. client has reached age of puberty
   b. persistent cross-sexual dressing
   c. at least two years' preoccupation with transforming their anatomy to that of the opposite sex
   d. persistent discomfort over anatomic sex

8. Psychological adjustment to sex reassignment
   a. is more favorable for female-to-male changes
   b. is more favorable for male-to-female changes
   c. has been shown to be poor regardless of direction of change
   d. has been shown to depend upon the quality of the surgical construction of sexual organs

9. Psychodynamic theorists view transsexualism as the result of
   a. overly permissive parents
   b. close mother-son relationships combined with empty father son relationships
   c. close father-son relationships combined with empty mother son relationships
   d. overly restrictive parents

10. Which of the following has been shown to result from viewing pornographic material?
    a. increased arousal in men but not in women
    b. increased arousal in women but not in men
    c. increased arousal in both men and women
    d. increase in deviant sexual practices for women but not for men

11. Experimental research by Donnerstien concluded that the greatest increase in the tendency to behave aggressively toward women occurred when men
    a. were shown aggressive-erotic pornography after being treated in a hostile manner
    b. were treated in a hostile manner by another couple
    c. were shown aggressive-erotic pornography after being treated in a neutral manner by another couple
    d. watched non-pornographic volent films after being provoked

12. Given that fewer than one in five rapes are actually reported it is estimated that _____ or more rapes occur in the United States each year.
    a. 75,000
    b. 90,000
    c. 200,000
    d. 375,000

13. Nicholas Groth and William Hobson have classified three basic kinds of rape:
    a. primary, secondary and tertiary
    b. homosexual, heterosexual and bisexual
    c. anger, power and sadistic
    d. date, acquaintance and stranger

139

14. Rape characterized by savage, unpremeditated attack triggered by hatred and resentment and often including coerced anal intercourse and fellatio is called

D
    a. violent rape
    b. sadistic rape
    c. power rape
    d. anger rape

15. Biological treatment approaches used with rapists

B
    a. assume that the rapist is motivated by internal conflicts
    b. have focused on protecting us from known rapists without much success
    c. are successful in eliminating the ability of rapists to engage in sex
    d. are generally agreed to be effective deterrents to rape

16. Methods of rape prevention

A
    a. are similar to recommendations to prevent other forms of crime
    b. include dressing conservatively
    c. are based on not sexually arousing men at parties
    d. have not been of much value in reducing the incidence of rape

17. Professional stripteasers and swimmers in revealing bathing suits

C
    a. meet the clinical criteria for exhibitionism
    b. do not meet the clinical criteria for exhibitionism because they are not attempting to sexually arouse the victim
    c. do not meet the clinical criteria for exhibitionism because the individuals they expose themselves to are not unsuspecting
    d. meet the clinical criteria for transvestic fetishism

18. The view that paraphilias are the result of some object or activity inadvertently becoming associated with sexual arousal, gaining the ability to elicit that arousal when the individual fantasizes about or acts out the paraphilias is associated with the _____ perspective.

B
    a. psychodynamic
    b. learning
    c. cognitive
    d. social learning

19. Female victims of childhood sexual abuse and incest show

A
    a. low self-esteem, self-blame, anger, coldness, and lack of trust
    b. more clearly developed sexualized behavior than females who were not abused sexually
    c. self-destructive behavior
    d. immediate negative consequences but not long-term effects of the abuse

20. Behavioral and cognitive therapies for paraphilias attempt

D
    a. to help the client to accept his behavior and fantasies
    b. to help the client adapt his behavior to minimize the effect it has on others
    c. to protect society from these individuals
    d. to disconnect arousal from the paraphiliac stimulus and reattach it to normal stimuli

21. Sexual reflexes in the excitement and orgasm stage
    a. occur in women but not in men
    b. occur in men but not in women
    c. are evidence of sexual dysfunction
    d. cannot be willed or forced

22. Sexual aversion disorder and hypoactive sexual desire disorder are both
    a. sexual desire disorders
    b. sexual arousal disorders
    c. orgasm disorders
    d. sexual pain disorders

23. A disorder involving involuntary spasm in the muscles of the vagina which makes sexual intercourse difficult or impossible is
    a. sexual aversion disorder
    b. female sexual arousal disorder
    c. dyspareunia
    d. vaginismus

24. Freud viewed premature ejaculation as symbolic of
    a. oral fixations
    b. hatred of women
    c. attachment to the father
    d. the electra complex

25. A technique to counter performance anxiety by teaching couples to engage in sexual stimulation exercises that do not require erection or vaginal lubrication is called
    a. self-spectatoring
    b. bibliotherapy
    c. sensate focus exercises
    d. mutual masturbation

TERMS AND CONCEPTS

TYING THINGS TOGETHER

1. As your text notes, the gay male community has changed its sexual practices in response to the risk of AIDS. Short of changing sexual orientation, what additional changes could be made to further reduce the risk of HIV infection? How might psychologists design treatment programs to encourage these changes? (NOTE: Answer this one well and there is a huge grant waiting for you at the National Institutes of Health when you finish graduate school.)

2. In the spring of 1989, Ted Bundy was executed for the murder of a young girl. Prior to his execution he confessed to a series of sexually motivated murders across the United states. He claimed that what made him do it was exposure to pornography. What do you think? Should we allow Ted Bundy's claim to sway our legal system an outlaw pornography? What about the First Amendment? Could we restrict access to those over 18? over 21? What should we do about pornographic material and what evidence can we cite to justify our decision?

3. Sex therapy was nonexistent at the time of the first Kinsey report. Since then it has shown dramatic growth and change that has benefitted many individuals suffering from sexual dysfunction. Your task is to write a brief essay about the nature of sex therapy in the twenty first century. Consider the changing cultural norms, should sexual dysfunctions be on the increase or decrease? What kinds of perspectives might have developed successful treatments not available today? What might treatment be like. Use your imagination, but base your fictional account on some current facts from this chapter.

ANSWERS

Lesson 1	Lesson 2	Lesson 3	Lesson 4
1 c	1 f	1 k	1 n
2 a	2 h	2 c	2 m
3 i	3 d	3 i	3 h
4 m	4 b	4 j	4 f
5 h	5 c	5 l	5 b
6 d	6 i	6 a	6 a
7 k	7 g	7 b	7 k
8 b	8 a	8 h	8 j
9 j	9 k	9 d	9 e
10 g	10 e	10 g	10 l
11 f	11 j	11 e	11 d
12 l		12 f	12 c
13 e			13 g
			14 i

True-False answers	Multiple-Choice answers
1 T	1 d
2 F	2 b
3 T	3 c
4 T	4 c
5 F	5 d
6 T	6 a
7 F	7 b
8 T	8 a
9 F	9 b
10 F	10 c
11 T	11 a
12 T	12 d
13 F	13 c
14 T	14 d
15 F	15 b
16 F	16 a
17 T	17 c
18 T	18 b
19 T	19 a
20 T	20 d
21 F	21 d
22 F	22 a
23 F	23 d
24 T	24 b
25 F	25 c

12 Schizophrenia and Delusional (Paranoid) Disorders

OVERVIEW

Have you ever felt like you've lost touch with reality? Instead of just feeling that way, some people do in fact lose touch with reality. These people suffer from schizophrenia. Chapter 12 "Schizophrenia and Delusional (Paranoid) Disorders" focuses on a disorder that afflicts between one and two percent of the world's population and is responsible for about half of the psychiatric hospitalizations.

You will find this a challenging chapter. It contains a very large number of new terms and concepts, all of which are necessary to give you a complete understanding of this very complex disorder. You will also find long and detailed sections on the theory and treatment of schizophrenia. These sections will be short on terms and concepts but long on detail. The theory section includes detailed discussion of research on the causes of schizophrenia. The treatment section provides an extensive analysis of treatment procedures. The unique combination of frequency and severity have made schizophrenia a heavily studied disorder. Schizophrenia's complexity has kept it more than a bit of a mystery.

Your chapter opens with a brief history of the disorder, tracing the roots of its discovery and diagnosis by Emil Kraepelin up to DSM-III-R. You will learn the "four A's" of schizophrenia. This will give you a sufficient understanding of the disorder to understand the following sections on prevalence of the disorder and phases of the disorder.

Next, your chapter takes a short detour. Two brief sections examine how schizophrenia differs from other psychoses and hallucinatory based disorders. These two sections should prepare you for an analysis of the diagnostic feature of schizophrenia.

The next section on the "Features of Schizophrenia" is a section which details the diagnostic features of schizophrenia. Table 12.1 (page 417 of your text) summarizes this information. This section identifies the major diagnostic criteria of schizophrenia and describes them in detail. A section on the types or sub-classifications recognized under DSM-III-R follows. Although they are not recognized under DSM-III-R, you chapter discusses three additional dimensions of schizophrenia, which are under consideration by researchers.

As with past chapters, sections discussing theories and therapies of the disorder follow. Each of the major theories of abnormal behavior discussed in Chapter 2 of your text have had a lot to say about both the theory and treatment of schizophrenia. Therefore, the sections on the "Theoretical Perspectives" and "Treatment" of schizophrenia are among the most detailed in the text.

145

The chapter finishes with a short section on delusional disorder. Delusional disorder is included in this chapter because of the similarity of its symptoms to paranoid schizophrenia.

CHAPTER OUTLINE, LESSONS & LEARNING OBJECTIVES

Lesson 1. The development of the concept of schizophrenia. (414-416)
HISTORY OF THE CONCEPT OF SCHIZOPHRENIA (414-416)
1. Describe the contributions of Emil Kraepelin, Eugen Bleuler, and Kurt Schneider to the concept of schizophrenia.
2. Describe the changes in the definition of schizophrenia from Kraepelin to the present day.

Lesson 2. Background to the diagnosis of schizophrenia. (416-419)
PREVALENCE OF SCHIZOPHRENIA (416-417)
3. Describe the prevalence of schizophrenia in the general population.
PHASES OF SCHIZOPHRENIA (417-418)
4. Describe the phasic nature of schizophrenia including the *prodromal phase*, *acute phase* or *acute episode*, and *residual phase*.
BRIEFER FORMS OF PSYCHOSIS (418)
5. Describe the differences between schizophrenia, brief reactive psychosis, and schizophreniform disorder.
SCHIZOPHRENIA-SPECTRUM DISORDERS (418-419)
6. Define the concept of schizophrenia-spectrum disorders and describe the differences between schizophrenia and schizoaffective disorder.

Lesson 3. Diagnostic features of schizophrenia. (419-424)
FEATURES OF SCHIZOPHRENIA (419-424)
7. Describe the disturbances in thought and speech that characterize schizophrenia.
8. Describe the recent psychophysical research on attention deficits in schizophrenia.
9. Describe perceptual disturbances in schizophrenia.
10. Describe emotional disturbances in schizophrenia.
11. Describe the disturbances in self-identity, volition, interpersonal behavior, and psychomotor behavior in schizophrenia.

Lesson 4. Types and dimensions of schizophrenia. (424-427)
TYPES OF SCHIZOPHRENIA (424-426)
12. Briefly summarize the historical changes in the classification of type of schizophrenia.
13. Describe the differences between the disorganized, catatonic, paranoid, and undifferentiated, and residual types of schizophrenia.
DIMENSIONS OF SCHIZOPHRENIA (426)
14. Describe the process-reactive dimension of schizophrenia, the positive-negative distinction of schizophrenic symptoms, and Type I - Type II distinction of schizophrenia.

Lesson 5. Theories of schizophrenic. (427-443)
THEORETICAL PERSPECTIVES (427-443)

15. Describe the psychodynamic, learning, biological, family, and sociocultural perspectives of schizophrenia.
16. Describe and evaluate the research on genetic factors, biochemical factors, viral infections, and brain damage.
17. Describe and evaluate the research on the diathesis-stress model of schizophrenia.

Lesson 6. Treatments for schizophrenia. (443-450)
TREATMENT (443-450)

18. Describe the biological, psychodynamic, learning-based, psychosocial-rehabilitation, and family-intervention treatments of schizophrenia.
19. Describe and evaluate the research on the effects and side effects of antipsychotic medication.

Lesson 7. The delusional (paranoid) disorder. (450-451)
DELUSIONAL (PARANOID) DISORDER (450-451)

20. Describe the characteristics of delusional (paranoid) disorder and describe the differences between it, paranoid schizophrenia, and paranoid personality disorder.

Mastering Lesson 1. The development of the concept of schizophrenia. (414-416)

This lesson consists of one short section tracing changes in the diagnosis of schizophrenia. There are five major different ways of diagnosing schizophrenia you need to know: Emil Kraepelin's, Eugen Bleuler's, Kurt Schneider's, DSM-III's, and DSM-III-R's. You do not need to know all of the details of DSM-III-R at this time. For each way of diagnosing schizophrenia, you will need to know the term used (it wasn't always schizophrenia), the major diagnostic criteria, and how this diagnosis changed the stringency of the diagnosis. The numbers of diagnosed schizophrenics changed as the diagnostic criteria became stricter or looser.

Match the following terms and concepts with the correct definition or description or explanation.

1. G dementia praecox
2. D Emil Kraepelin
3. H Eugen Bleuler
4. I first-rank symptoms
5. A four A's of schizophrenia
6. B Kurt Schneider
7. C schizophrenic affect
8. E schizophrenic ambivalence
9. E schizophrenic associations
10. K schizophrenic autism
11. J second-rank symptoms

a. associations, affect, ambivalence, and autism
b. developed first-rank - second-rank distinction
c. emotional response become flat or inappropriate
d. first to label the schizophrenic behavior pattern as a medical syndrome
e. holding strong and opposing feelings toward other persons
f. ideas shift from one topic to another with linkages between topics
g. premature loss of one's mental abilities
h. renamed dementia praecox schizophrenia
i. symptoms central to the diagnosis of and unique to schizophrenia
j. symptoms schizophrenia shares with other disorders
k. withdrawal into a fantasy world without logic

147

Mastering Lesson 2. Background to the diagnosis of schizophrenia. (416-419)

This lesson represents a short detour. There are four brief sections. The first discusses how prevalent schizophrenia is; the second examines three phases schizophrenia goes through; the third shows how other psychoses differ from schizophrenia; and the fourth examines how other hallucinatory disorders differ from schizophrenia. These last two sections tell you what schizophrenia isn't in preparation for what it is. This information could have been discussed either before or after the diagnostic criteria were examined. We suspect that your authors chose to discuss them here so they wouldn't get lost in what follows. Yes, it is going to get deep very soon.

Match the following terms and concepts with the correct definition or description or explanation.

1. H 1-2%
2. E acute episode
3. C acute phase
4. B brief reactive psychosis
5. D prodromal phase
6. E residual phase
7. A schizoaffective disorders
8. G schizophreniform disorder

a. a "mixed bag" of psychotic behaviors and mood disturbance
b. a psychotic episode in response to a traumatic event
c. period of active schizophrenic symptoms with gradual onset
d. period of deterioration leading to active schizophrenia
e. rapid onset of schizophrenic symptoms
f. return to prodromal like behavior following the acute phase
g. schizophrenic symptoms for a period less than six months
h. the prevalence of schizophrenic episodes in the general population

Mastering Lesson 3. Diagnostic features of schizophrenia. (419-424)

In a mere five pages, you are going to encounter over 20 new key terms and concepts. The section on the "Features of Schizophrenia" details the diagnostic features of schizophrenia. Table 12.1 (page 417 of your text) summarizes the information contained in this section. You need to know the information in Table 12.1 6 in detail. Your chapter also identifies and discusses by name a number of delusions, speech disorders, and hallucinations. We have included those names in the matching test below and the list of key terms and concepts. You need to know this information also.

Then comes the problem of deficits in attention in schizophrenia. Do not ignore the section on pages 421-422 on "Event-Related Potentials" just because it contains no key terms. This section summarizes research which your instructor may find quite interesting. (For interesting, you might read "is likely to ask questions about.")

Any time you are confronted with research to remember, you should make up a chart summarizing the research. RAH makes charts for each study he is trying to remember. Each chart contains three rows. The top row consists of a series of boxes. Each box contains a description of each group or condition in the study or experiment. Below each box on the first row, RAH summarizes the results for each group in another box. The third row consists of brief summary statements of the results and what they mean. A good chart will contain more words than the text uses to describe the experiment. Although this may seem time consuming, you will be able to remember the procedure and results of the study.

Lesson 3 may take you only a few minutes to read but hours to master.

Match the following terms and concepts with the correct definition or description or explanation.

1. S blocking
2. W clanging
3. M deficiencies in orienting response
4. I deficits in attention
5. E delusion of being controlled
6. G delusion of persecution
7. E delusion of reference
8. N delusions
9. A delusion of grandeur
10. K disturbances in the content of thought
11. Q disturbances in the form of thought
12. O emotional disturbances
13. U event-related potentials
14. V eye movement dysfunctions
15. Z hallucinations
16. H hypervigilant
17. L impaired level of functioning
18. Y loss of ego boundaries
19. T neologisms
20. X orienting response
21. P perceptual disturbances
22. R perseveration
23. C thought broadcasting
24. J thought disorder
25. B thought insertion
26. D thought withdrawal

a. "I am on a mission from God to save the world"
b. "martians are putting ideas in my head"
c. "martians can hear me thinking"
d. "martians drained the secrets of the universe from my brain"
e. "people on television are talking about me"
f. "someone is controlling by actions"
g. "someone is spying on me"
h. a schizophrenic's acute sensitivity to extraneous sounds
i. a schizophrenic's inability to ignore irrelevant distracting stimuli
j. another name for disturbances in the form or structure of thought
k. delusions of persecution and thought insertion, for example
l. difficulty in holding a conversation or keeping a job
m. failure of schizophrenics to show normal orienting response
n. false and illogical beliefs which cannot be disconfirmed
o. flattened and inappropriate affect
p. hallucinations of any of the five senses
q. impaired ability to think and speak meaningfully
r. inappropriate and persistent repetition of the same thought
s. involuntary interruptions of speech
t. making up words with little or no meaning
u. schizophrenics have abnormal brain wave patterns to stimuli
v. schizophrenics have difficulty visually tracking moving objects
w. stringing words together which rhyme without meaning
x. the automatic psychophysiological responses to incoming stimuli
y. the failure of persons to recognize that they are unique individuals
z. the perception of an event in absence of external stimulation

Mastering Lesson 4. Types and dimensions of schizophrenia. (424-427)

This lesson consists of two brief sections. The first discusses types or sub-classifications of schizophrenia recognized by DSM-III-R. There are five. The second section examines three dimensions of schizophrenia, which are not recognized under DSM-III-R, but are under consideration by researchers.

Match the following terms and concepts with the correct definition or description or explanation.

1. J prognosis
2. H premorbid adjustment
3. A waxy flexibility
4. K Type I
5. L Type II
6. N process schizophrenia
7. M reactive schizophrenia
8. E negative symptoms
9. I positive symptoms
10. F catatonic type
11. C disorganized type
12. B paranoid type
13. D residual type
14. G undifferentiated type

a. the adoption of a fixed posture
b. complex and systematic delusion of grandeur and persecution
c. confused behavior, vivid hallucinations, and disorganized delusions
d. shows signs of previous schizophrenic episodes
e. behavioral deficits or the absence of normal behavior
f. markedly impaired motor behavior showing stupor and agitation
g. do not meet the specifications of other types
h. level of functioning before the acute phase
i. excessive or distorted behavior
j. the predicted outcome of a disorder
k. favorable response to antipsychotic medication
l. poor response to antipsychotic medication
m. schizophrenia with clearly identified onset
n. schizophrenia with no clearly identified onset

Mastering Lesson 5. Theories of schizophrenic. (427-443)

As the title indicates, this lesson covers theories of schizophrenia. Each major theory of abnormal behavior discussed in Chapter 2 of your text has something to say about schizophrenia. Along with a brief discussion of each theory is an extensive discussion of research concerning each theoretical perspective. This is particularly true about the section on "Biological Perspectives" which devotes considerable attention to research. Therefore, the section on the "Theoretical Perspectives" is long (17 pages) and very detailed. This section is short on key terms and concepts and long on research.

As we discussed before, you should take extensive notes on each study or experiment discussed in your text so that you can remember what was done and what was discovered. We would bet that your instructor will ask you about the twin study whose results are summarized in Figure 12.2 on page 430 ; the adoption studies covered on pages 431-432; and the studies of HR children of pages 433-435. If you're beginning to feel like we are telling you to know everything, we are. This is important stuff. If we were taking a test over this material, we would have about 10 pages of reading notes on the research discussed in this section. If you are making charts of the research you read about, you will find that some of the studies discussed in this section will require more than one chart.

Match the following terms and concepts with the correct definition or description or explanation.

1. P primary narcissism
2. O distinct heterogeneity model
3. N monogenic model
4. M multifactorial-polygenic model
5. L diathesis-stress model
6. K markers
7. J HR children
8. H vulnerability factors
9. I protective factors
10. G dopamine theory
11. F viral theory
12. E schizophrenogenic mother
13. D double-bind communications
14. C communication deviance
15. B expressed emotion
16. A institutionalization syndrome

a. a pattern of passive and dependent behavior in hospitalized persons
b. negative emotion expressed toward a schizophrenic family member
c. a pattern of vagueness and blurred meaning in parental communication
d. two mutually incompatible meanings in a single message
e. a cold, aloof, domineering mother who reduces self-esteem and independence
f. schizophrenia results from a slow-acting virus attacking the brain
g. schizophrenia results from excessive reactivity of receptors in the brain
h. factors that increase risk among HR children
i. factors that decrease risk among HR children
j. children with a high risk of developing schizophrenia
k. identifiable factors which differentiate HR children from others
l. genetic disposition that is released by stressful environments
m. interactive effects of multiple genes, prenatal, and postnatal factors
n. there is a single gene for schizophrenia
o. schizophrenia is a number of disorders, some of which are genetic
p. the ego overwhelmed by id impulses reverts to early oral stage

Mastering Lesson 6. Treatments for schizophrenia. (443-450)

This lesson covers treatment of schizophrenia. Each theory of abnormal behavior discussed in Chapter 2, except the cognitive approach, has had something to say about the treatment of schizophrenia. Your chapter discusses all of them but focuses on biologically based therapy, behaviorally based therapy, and socio-culturally based therapy. The biological approach has emphasized the use of antipsychotic drugs. Although these drugs provide relief from schizophrenic symptoms, they do not cure the disease and have serious side effects. Behavioral approach has emphasized training in social skills through modeling, operant conditioning, and token economies. This approach has been successful in improving social skills of schizophrenics. The socio-cultural approach has emphasized family intervention programs targeting the families of schizophrenics. Despite the severity of schizophrenia, training families to respond to schizophrenics differently can provide relatively effective treatment.

The focus of this section is not on terms and concepts. Rather the focus of this section is on describing how the therapy is done, how effective it is, and what drawbacks might exist for the therapy. Therefore, the list of terms and concepts for this section is short. Above and beyond the terms and concepts, there is considerable information to learn.

Match the following terms and concepts with the correct definition or description or explanation.

1. _B_ neuroleptics   a. side effect of long term use of antipsychotic drugs
2. _A_ tardive dyskinesia   b. major tranquilizers

Mastering Lesson 7. The delusional (paranoid) disorder. (450-451)

The chapter finishes with and this lesson covers a short section on delusional disorder. Delusional disorder is included in this chapter because of the similarity of its symptoms to paranoid schizophrenia.

Match the following terms and concepts with the correct definition or description or explanation.

1. _A_ delusional disorders   a. disorders characterized by delusions without the confused or jumbled thinking of schizophrenia
2. _C_ erotomanic type
3. _F_ grandiose type   b. delusions involving physical defects and disease
4. _E_ jealous type   c. delusions that a famous person is in love with you
5. _D_ persecutory type   d. delusions that one is being conspired against
6. _B_ somatic type   e. delusions that one's lover is unfaithful
     f. delusions that you have special mystical powers

PRACTICE EXAM

Exam 1. (true-false)

Indicate whether each of the following statements is **True** or **False**. Question numbers correspond to learning objectives from which the questions were drawn.

1. _F_ Kurt Schneider was the first to identify the disorder of schizophrenia.
2. _F_ The adoption of DSM-III-R criteria has increased the number of cases diagnosed as schizophrenic.
3. _F_ Schizophrenics occupy more than one-half of the psychiatric hospital beds in the United States.
4. _F_ The gradual onset of schizophrenia is called an acute episode.
5. _T_ A schizophreniform disorder is longer than a brief reactive psychosis.
6. _F_ Schizoaffective disorder is more severe than schizophrenia in terms of expected outcome.
7. _T_ Clanging is a type of thought disorder.
8. _T_ Schizophrenics show greater P300 ERPs than normal individuals.
9. _T_ Hallucinations are the most common perceptual disturbance in schizophrenia.
10. _T_ Reduced emotional responsiveness is called "blunt affect."
11. _T_ Schizophrenics may adopt and hold a rigid posture for extended periods of time.
12. _F_ In DSM-III-R, there are four types of schizophrenia.
13. _F_ Hallucinations are most active in catatonic schizophrenia.
14. _T_ Rapid onset schizophrenia is sometimes called reactive.
15. _T_ Concordance for schizophrenia increases as genetic similarity increases.
16. _T_ A "high-risk" child is the adopted child of a schizophrenic mother.
17. _T_ The diathesis-stress model suggests that stress alone produces schizophrenia

T (18.) F Behaviorally based treatments have improved the behavior of "hard-core" schizophrenics who were unresponsive to medication.

19. T A major problem of using antipsychotic drugs is that they have serious side effects.

F (20.) T The delusional (paranoid) disorder is characterized by the presence of hallucinations.

Exam 2 (multiple-choice)

Select the single, best answer for each question. Question numbers correspond to learning objectives from which the questions were drawn.

1. Who was the person who first characterized schizophrenia as a disorder of the "four A's?"
   a. Bleuler
   b. Freud
   c. Kraepelin
   d. Schneider

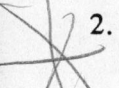

2. Whose theory of schizophrenia was heavily influenced by psychodynamic theory?
   a. Bleuler's
   b. Kraepelin's
   c. Schneider's
   d. Vincente's

3. Approximately ____ of the world's population will have a schizophrenic episode.
   a. 1-2%
   b. 5-10%
   c. 25%
   d. 50%

4. Which of the following is in the correct order?
   a. acute phase, prodromal phase, residual phase
   b. acute episode, residual phase, prodromal phase
   c. residual phase, prodromal phase, acute phase
   d. prodromal phase, acute phase, residual phase

5. A person must show abnormal behavior for how long before they are diagnosed as schizophrenic?
   a. 30 days
   b. 3 months
   c. 6 months
   d. 1 year

6. A person with schizoaffective disorder will show which of the following symptoms not usually present in schizophrenia?
   a. persistent delusions
   b. persistent hallucination
   c. persistent manic-depression
   d. persistent waxy flexibility

7. What is the inappropriately and persistently repeating the same words or train or thought?
   a. thought broadcasting
   b. thought withdrawal
   c. perseveration
   d. blocking

8. Schizophrenics are
   a. more likely to be distracted by irrelevant stimuli than normals
   b. less likely to be distracted by irrelevant stimuli than normals
   c. more likely to ignore relevant stimuli than normals
   d. more likely to perseverate on relevant stimuli than normals

9. Hallucinations are defined as images _____ in the _____ of external stimulation.
   a. perceived; absence
   b. perceived; presence
   c. not perceived; absence
   d. not perceived; presence

10. Schizophrenics, in general, experience _____ range of emotions than normal persons.
    a. a narrower
    b. a wider
    c. the same
    d. a different

11. Which of the following statements with regard to schizophrenia is true?
    a. Schizophrenics develop stronger interpersonal attachment than normals.
    b. Schizophrenics are more confused about their personal identify than normals.
    c. Schizophrenics show more initiative than normals.
    d. Schizophrenics have stronger ego boundaries than normals.

12. Which of the following is not one of the types of schizophrenia recognized by DSM-III-R?
    a. simple
    b. disorganized
    c. undifferentiated
    d. residual

13. Delusions of grandeur are most present in which type of schizophrenia?
    a. disorganized
    b. residual
    c. simple
    d. paranoid

14. The Type I - Type II distinction is similar to the _____ distinction.
    a. reactive - process
    b. simple - undifferentiated
    c. positive - negative symptom
    d. genetic - behavioral

15. If one twin of a pair of monozygotic (genetically identical) twins develops schizophrenia, what is the likelihood that other twin will develop schizophrenia?
    a. less than 10%
    b. 40% - 50%
    c. 75%-80%
    d. more than 90%

16. If a child is placed into a adoptive or foster home with a schizophrenic parent, this child _____ to develop schizophrenia than a child placed into a home without a schizophrenic parent.
    a. is less likely
    b. is more likely
    c. is just as likely
    d. is we don't know how likely

17. Birth trauma among _____ children _____ the likelihood that they will develop schizophrenia.
    a. LR; increases
    b. HR; increases
    c. LR; decreases
    d. HR; decreases

18. Which type of therapy is least effective, in fact practically useless, in the treatment of schizophrenics?
    a. behavioral
    b. biological
    c. psychodynamic
    d. family intervention

19. Schizophrenics who are responsive to antipsychotic drugs
    a. can be taken off the drugs with no ill effect.
    b. will continue to show improvement if treated with placebo drugs.
    c. only show improvement if they continue to take the drugs.
    d. show fewer side effects than those who are not responsive.

20. The most common type of delusional disorder is the _____ type.
    a. erotomanic
    b. grandiose
    c. jealous
    d. persecutory

155

TERMS AND CONCEPTS

Lesson 1
dementia praecox (414)
Emil Kraepelin (414)
Eugen Bleuler (415)
first-rank symptoms (416)
four A's of schizophrenia (415)
Kurt Schneider (416)
schizophrenic affect (415)
schizophrenic ambivalence (415)
schizophrenic associations (415)
schizophrenic autism (415)
second-rank symptoms (416)

Lesson 2
1-2% (416)
acute episode (417)
acute phase (418)
brief reactive psychosis (418)
prodromal phase (418)
residual phase (418)
schizoaffective disorders (418)
schizophreniform disorder (418)

Lesson 3
blocking (420)
clanging (420)
deficiencies in orienting response (421)
deficits in attention (420)
delusion of being controlled (419)
delusion of persecution (419)
delusion of reference (419)
delusions (419)
delusion of grandeur (419)
disturbances in the content of thought (419)
disturbances in the form of thought (420)
emotional disturbances (424)
event-related potentials (421)
eye movement dysfunctions (421)
hallucinations (422)
hypervigilant (421)
impaired level of functioning (419)
loss of ego boundaries (424)
negative symptoms (421)
neologisms (420)
orienting response (421)
perceptual disturbances (422)
perseveration (420)
positive symptoms (421)
thought broadcasting (419)
thought disorder (420)
thought insertion (419)
thought withdrawal (419)

Lesson 4
catatonic type (425)
disorganized type (424)
negative symptoms (427)
paranoid type (426)
positive symptoms (427)
premorbid adjustment (426)
process schizophrenia (426)
prognosis (426)
reactive schizophrenia (426)
residual type (424)
Type I (427)
Type II (427)
undifferentiated type (424)
waxy flexibility (425)

Lesson 5
communication deviance (440)
diathesis-stress model (433)
distinct heterogeneity model (432)
dopamine theory (436)
double-bind communications (440)
expressed emotion (441)
HR children (433)
institutionalization syndrome (442)
markers (433)
monogenic model (432)
multifactorial-polygenic model (432)
primary narcissism (428)
protective factors (435)
schizophrenogenic mother (440)
viral theory (437)
vulnerability factors (435)

TYING THINGS TOGETHER

1. Identify the key diagnostic criteria you would use to differentiate delusional (paranoid) disorder from paranoid personality disorder from paranoid schizophrenia.

2. Identify the key diagnostic criteria you would use to differentiate schizophrenia from schizotypal personality disorder from schizoaffective disorder.

3. Studies of MZ and DZ twins raised together and apart prove that genes and environment contribute to the development of schizophrenia. Using the research discussed in your text show that this statement is true. Why does this evidence support the diathesis-stress model?

4. Why would the Type I - Type II distinction be important if it were true?

ANSWERS

<u>Lesson 1</u>
1 g
2 d
3 h
4 i
5 a
6 b
7 c
8 e
9 f
10 k
11 j

<u>Lesson 2</u>
1 h
2 e
3 c
4 b
5 d
6 f
7 a
8 g

<u>Lesson 3</u>
1 s
2 w
3 m
4 i
5 f
6 g
7 e
8 n
9 a
10 k
11 q
12 o
13 u
14 v
15 z
16 h
17 l
18 y
19 t
20 x
21 p
22 r
23 c
24 j
25 b
26 d

<u>Lesson 4</u>
1 j
2 h
3 a
4 k
5 l
6 n
7 m
8 e
9 i
10 f
11 c
12 b
13 d
14 g

<u>Lesson 5</u>
1 p
2 o
3 n
4 m
5 l
6 k
7 j
8 h
9 i
10 g
11 f
12 e
13 d
14 c
15 b
16 a

<u>Lesson 6</u>
1 b
2 a

<u>Lesson 7</u>
1 a
2 c
3 f
4 e
5 d
6 b

True-False	Multiple-Choice
answers	answers
1 F	1 a
2 F	2 b
3 T	3 a
4 F	4 d
5 T	5 c
6 F	6 c
7 F	7 c
8 F	8 a
9 T	9 a
10 T	10 a
11 T	11 b
12 F	12 a
13 F	13 d
14 T	14 a
15 T	15 b
16 T	16 c
17 F	17 b
18 T	18 c
19 T	19 c
20 F	20 d

13 Organic Disorders and Abnormal Behavior

OVERVIEW

This chapter provides the briefest of introductions into the relationship between physical disorders of the brain and abnormal behavior. You will begin to feel a bit like a medical student because throughout the chapter you will need to know three things. The name of an organic disease or disorder, the physical conditions which produce or cause it, and the pattern of behaviors or symptoms for that disorder.

Your chapter begins with, and the first lesson covers, an examination of two major classes of organic disorders recognized by DSM-III-R, the organic mental disorder and the organic mental syndromes. The diagnostic distinction DSM-III-R makes between these two types of disorder provides background for the rest of the chapter.

The next three sections of the text, "Delirium," "Amnestic Syndrome," and "Dementias" cover disorders which are grouped by symptom similarity. The next five sections group disorders first by the region of the brain affected and then by the source of the organic damage.

Two brief sections on disorder caused by nutritional deficits and endocrine malfunction follow. The chapter ends with an examination of epilepsy. As you will discover, epilepsy is not a single disorder but a group of disorders. Different types of epilepsy have different causes, different symptoms, and effect different portions of the brain.

CHAPTER OUTLINE, LESSONS & LEARNING OBJECTIVES

Lesson 1. Distinguishing organic mental disorders from organic mental syndromes. (456-459)

ORGANIC MENTAL DISORDERS AND SYNDROMES (456-459)

1. Describe the features of organic mental disorders.
2. Describe the problems involved in diagnosing organic mental disorders.
3. Describe the differences between organic mental disorders and organic mental syndromes.
4. Describe the features of organic mental syndromes.

Lesson 2. Delirium and amnestic syndrome. (459-461)

DELIRIUM (459-460)

5. Identify, define, and describe the causes of *delirium*.

AMNESTIC SYNDROME (460-461)

6. Describe the features and causes of amnestic syndrome.
7. Summarize the origins and features of Korsakoff's syndrome.

161

Lesson 3. Organic dementias. (461-469)
DEMENTIAS (461-469)
8. Discuss whether or not dementias are a normal feature of aging.
9a. Describe the relationship between depression and memory loss among the elderly.
9b. Describe cognitive-behavioral approaches to treating depression among the elderly.
10. Describe the features and incidence of Alzheimer's disease.
11. Describe the impact that Alzheimer's disease can have on the family.
12. Describe the hypotheses for the causes of Alzheimer's disease.
13. Describe the features of multi-infarct dementia.
14. Describe the features of Pick's disease.

Lesson 4. Diseases of the Basal Ganglia. (470-472)
DISEASES OF THE BASAL GANGLIA (470-472)
15. Describe the features, origins, and treatment of Parkinson's disease.
16. Describe the features of Huntington's disease.
17. Describe the genetic transmission of Huntington's disease.

Lesson 5. Diseases of the cortex. (472-475)
INFECTIONS OF THE BRAIN (472-473)
18. Describe the features of encephalitis, meningitis, neurosyphilis, and AIDS dementia complex.
BRAIN TRAUMA (473-474)
19. Describe the possible effects of concussions, contusions, and lacerations of the brain.
CEREBROVASCULAR DISORDERS (474-475)
20. Identify, define, and describe the effects of strokes and cerebral hemorrhages.
BRAIN TUMORS
21. Define and describe the effects of brain tumors.

Lesson 6. Nutritional deficiencies and endocrine disorders. (475-476)
NUTRITIONAL DEFICIENCIES (475-476)
22. Define and describe the effects of pellagra and beriberi.
ENDOCRINE DISORDERS (476)
23. Identify, define, and describe the features of disorders caused by thyroid and adrenal dysfunctions.

Lesson 7. Epilepsy. (476-479) *Early signs – wandering, staring spells,*
EPILEPSY (476-479) *memory gaps, bedwetting, violent muscle spasms in sleep*
nocturnal tongue-biting.
24. Discuss the stigma attached to epilepsy.
25. Define the various types of epilepsy.
26. Outline the myths and facts of epilepsy discussed in your text.
27. Describe the treatments for epilepsy.

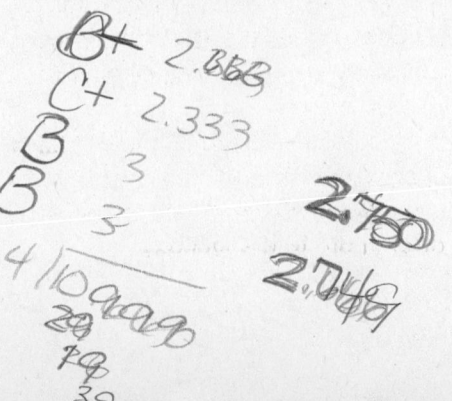

162

Mastering Lesson 1. Distinguishing organic mental disorders from organic mental syndromes. (456-459)

The chapter begins by presenting you with a definition of and diagnostic problems with organic mental <u>disorders</u>. The features of organic mental disorders are summarized by Table 13.1 (page 457). The chapter continues with by presenting a definition of organic mental <u>syndromes</u>, the features for which are in Table 13.2 (page 458). We confess that we have trouble keeping the difference between them straight. Therefore, we would suggest asking your instructor to explain what he wants you to know on this issue. The two types of disorders are coded on different axes of DSM-III-R and we have asked you to know that below.

Match the following terms and concepts with the correct definitions or description or explanation.

1. _A_ agnosia
2. _B_ organic mental disorders
3. _C_ organic mental syndromes

  a. an inability to see
  b. disorders associated with temporary or permanent brain damage
  c. disorders believed to be caused by organic disorders affecting the brain

Mastering Lesson 2. Delirium and amnestic syndrome. (459-461)

Delirium and amnesia are two relative frequently occurring disorders, particularly among those who abuse drugs. Table 13.3 (page 459) summarizes the features of the three levels of delirium and should be memorized. For each of the disorders in this lesson, you will need to know its name (and any alternative names), its causes, and its symptoms.

Match the following terms and concepts with the correct definition or description or explanation.

1. _F_ alcohol amnestic disorder
2. _D_ amnestic syndrome
3. _C_ ataxia
4. _E_ delirium
5. _B_ delirium tremens
6. _A_ Korsakoff's syndrome

  a. another name of alcohol amnestic disorder
  b. delirium caused by abrupt withdrawal from alcohol
  c. difficulty in maintaining one's balance while walking
  d. dramatic decline in memory which is not due to a delirium or dementia
  e. severe difficulty in concentrating and psychological disorganization
  f. short and long term memory loss due to chronic alcohol abuse

Mastering Lesson 3. Organic dementias. (461-469)

Dementias are significant declines in memory and general intellectual functioning. In this the longest and most detailed section in this chapter, your text examines and identifies different types of organic dementia, their origin, and their symptoms. Before doing so, your chapter examines two related issues, memory loss and depression in the elderly.

Your chapter discusses three major types of dementia, Alzheimer's disease, multi-infarct dementia, and Pick's disease. The most prevalent of these is Alzheimer's disease. Therefore, your text covers Alzheimer's disease more thoroughly than any other topic in the chapter. In addition,

163

you chapter examines the problems presented for the families of Alzheimer's victims. Again, you will need to be able to identify these disorders, describe the causes or theories of these disorders, and the symptoms of these disorders.

Match the following terms and concepts with the correct definition or description or explanation.

1. _H_ Alzheimer's disease
2. _G_ aphasia
3. _A_ dementia
4. _B_ Global Deterioration Scale or GDS
5. _E_ multi-infarct dementia or MID
6. _H_ Pick's Disease
7. _D_ presenile demential
8. _C_ senile dementia

a. an abnormal and significant decline in intellectual functioning
b. compares normal decline with decline due to Alzheimer's
c. dementia after age 65
d. dementia before age 65
e. dementia caused by the presence of Pick's bodies in nerve cells.
f. dementia caused by small repeated strokes
g. loss of the ability to speak or understand speech
h. severe dementia caused by neuritic plaques and neurofibril tangles

Mastering Lesson 4. Diseases of the Basal Ganglia. (470-472)

This is the first section in which disorders are grouped by the location of organic damage. The two diseases in this section, Parkinson's and Huntington's, are both disorders of the basal ganglia, a group of neuron cell bodies that lie beneath the cortex. The basal ganglia helps control and coordinate sequences of movement. You will need to pay particular attention to the problems of genetic transmission associated with Huntington's disease.

Match the following terms and concepts with the correct definitions or description or explanation.

1. _A_ basal ganglia
2. _B_ Huntington's disease
3. _C_ Parkinson's disease

a. group of cell bodies which lie under the cortex and control motor behavior
b. involuntary jerky dance-like movements, often combined with depression
c. shaking, tremors, abnormal posture, and lack of control over movements

164

Mastering Lesson 5. Diseases of the cortex. (472-475)

This lesson covers four very brief sections of your text. All of them examine ways that disease can effect the cerebral cortex. Each section examines a different source for brain damage or disease, viral infections, head injury, vascular accident, and the development of tumors. Again, you need to know the disease, cause, and effect triad.

Match the following terms and concepts with the correct definition or description or explanation.

1. _L_ AIDS dementia complex
2. _F_ brain tumors
3. _G_ cerebral hemorrhage
4. _B_ cerebrovascular disorder
5. _D_ concussion
6. _E_ contusion
7. _I_ encephalitis
8. _K_ general paresis
9. _C_ laceration
10. _J_ meningitis
11. _H_ neurosyphilis
12. _A_ stroke

a. brain damage due to the blockage of a blood vessel
b. brain disorder caused by vascular accident
c. brain injury caused by a foreign object piercing the skull
d. brain trauma caused by a hard blow producing loss of consciousness
e. bruising of the brain caused by a hard blow
f. cause damage by exerting pressure on the brain
g. damage produced by blood vessels rupturing, causing blood to leak onto the brain
h. general term to describe the effects of syphilis on the brain
i. inflammation of the brain
j. inflammation of the membranes that cover the spinal cord and brain
k. mental deterioration caused by syphilitic infection
l. progressive decline in mental and motor function due to the AIDS virus

Mastering Lesson 6. Nutritional deficiencies and endocrine disorders. (475-476)

This is a very short lesson covering two sections. The first covers how niacin and thiamine deficiencies lead to pellagra and beriberi, respectively. The second covers how over- and under-activity in the thyroid and adrenal glands effects behavior.

Match the following terms and concepts with the correct definition or description or explanation.

1. _A_ Addison's disease
2. _G_ beriberi
3. _E_ cretinism
4. _B_ Cushing's syndrome
5. _D_ hyperthyroidism
6. _C_ hypothyroidism
7. _H_ pellagra
8. _F_ thyroxin

a. caused by decreased activity in the adrenal cortex
b. caused by overactivity of adrenal cortex
c. secretion of too little thyroxin
d. secretion of too much thyroxin
e. stunted growth and mental retardation produced by hypothyroidism
f. substance secreted by the thyroid gland
g. thiamine deficiency producing memory loss, insomnia, and lack of appetite
h. vitamin B deficiency producing anxiety, depression, and memory loss

Mastering Lesson 7. Epilepsy. (476-479)

The last section of and lesson for this chapter covers epilepsy. Epilepsy is <u>not</u> a single disorder or disease; rather epilepsy is the name given to a group of disorders. The "epilepsies" are disorders in which the electrical rhythms of brain are disturbed. This disturbance leads to seizures and/or losses of consciousness.

The key to understanding this lesson is to identify and define the various types of epilepsies, their symptoms and causes. Because epilepsy is misunderstood, your text presents a table of "Myths and Facts about Epilepsy" (page 478); you need to know this information.

Match the following terms and concepts with the correct definition or description or explanation.

1. _C_ acquired epilepsy
2. _A_ epilepsy
3. _F_ *grand mal* seizure
4. _D_ idiopathic epilepsy
5. _E_ *petit mal* epilepsy
6. _B_ tonic-clonic epilepsy

a. disturbances in the electrical patterns of the brain
b. epilepsy characterized by *grand mal* seizure
c. epilepsy due to known causes
d. epilepsy for unknown causes
e. involuntary lapses in consciousness without motor involvement
f. loss of consciousness, convulsive and jerking movements, and memory loss

PRACTICE EXAM

Exam 1. (true-false)

Indicate whether each of the following statements is **True** or **False**. Question numbers correspond to learning objectives from which the questions were drawn.

1. _T_ An organic mental disorder is associated with temporary or permanent dysfunction of the brain.
2. _F_ If two persons have damage to the same area of the brain, they will have identical symptoms.
3. _F_ Organic mental syndromes are coded on Axis I of DSM-III-R.
4. _T_ Amnestic syndrome is an organic mental syndrome.
5. _T_ Abrupt withdrawal from chronic alcohol abuse can induce an organic mental syndrome.
6. _F_ Amnestic syndrome is characterized by loss of memory due to dementia.
7. _F_ Alcohol amnestic syndrome is only produced by alcohol abuse.
8. _F_ Dementia is a normal part of the aging process.
9. _F_ Memory loss is the major cause of depression in the elderly.
10. _T_ Alzheimer's disease accounts for about 75% of all dementias.
11. _T_ Most persons suffering from Alzheimer's disease eventually require around the clock attention.
12. _T_ Alzheimer's victims show abnormally high levels of aluminum in their brains.
13. _T_ The onset of multi-infarct dementia is more rapid than an Alzheimer's dementia.
14. _T_ Pick's disease can only be differentiated from Alzheimer's at autopsy.
15. _F_ Parkinson's disease can be cured by administration of L-dopa.
16. _T_ Huntington's disease involves the deterioration of neurons producing GABA in the basal ganglia.

166

17. F Huntington's disease is a sex-linked genetic disease only going from father to son.
18. T If left untreated, syphilis will infect the brain.
19. T Contusions of the brain can produce permanent damage.
20. T A common effect of a stroke is the loss of speech.
21. F Only cancerous brain tumors produce organic mental syndromes.
22. T Pellagra can produce loss of memory, hallucinations, and delusions.
23. T Addison's disease is characterized by weight loss and low blood pressure.
24. T Physicians may diagnose epilepsy as a seizure disorder to avoid stigma for their patients.
25. F The most severe form of epilepsy is idiopathic epilepsy.
26. F Male epileptics may commit rape during a seizure.
27. T Surgery can cure some epileptics.

Exam 2 (multiple-choice)

Select the single, best answer for each question. Question numbers correspond to learning objectives from which the questions were drawn.

1. An organic mental disorder has which of the following features?
    a. loss of memory for recent events
    b. depression following loss
    c. savant-like intellectual performance
    d. all of the above are features

2. Which of the following is one of the difficulties in diagnosing organic mental disorders?
    a. neurological symptoms can look like psychosocial symptoms
    b. CAT scans will not detect all neurological problems
    c. social support can reduce the severity of organic problems
    d. all of the above are difficulties

3. A person who is suffering from delirium due to a temporary infection is suffering from which of the following?
    A
    a. an organic mental disorder
    b. an organic mental syndrome
    c. delirium tremens
    d. Korsakoff's syndrome

4. Prominent and recurrent hallucinations is a feature of which organic mental syndrome?
    B
    a. organic delusion syndrome
    b. organic hallucinosis
    c. organic anxiety syndrome
    d. organic personality syndrome

5. Which of the following is one of the features of severe delirium?
    C
    a. apprehension
    b. fear
    c. panic
    d. myocardia

167

6. Amnestic syndrome is often of a consequence of which of the following?
   a. alcohol abuse
   b. drug abuse
   c. head trauma
   d. viral infection

7. Which of the following is another name for alcohol amnestic syndrome?
   a. Alzheimer's syndrome
   b. Korsakoff's syndrome
   c. Wernicke's syndrome
   d. Vitamin hypertaxia

8. Senile dementia begins after age ____.
   a. 45
   b. 55
   c. 65
   d. 75

9. What is the best way to characterize depression in the elderly?
   a. it is a minor problem for a few
   b. it is major problem for a few
   c. it is a minor problem for many
   d. it is a major problem for many

10. The diagnosis of Alzheimer's disease depends upon finding which of the following?
    a. abnormal loss of memory
    b. inability to manage everyday tasks
    c. neuritic plagues and neurofibrillary tangles
    d. basal ganglia atrophy

11. Medicare, the federal system of health care for the elderly, covers what percent of the nursing home health care costs of an Alzheimer's victim?
    a. 0%
    b. 25%
    c. 50%
    d. 80%

12. The son or daughter of an Alzheimer's victim is ____ likely to get Alzheimer's as a person whose parent does or did not have Alzheimer's.
    a. less
    b. no more
    c. 4 times more
    d. 10 times more

13. Multi-infarct dementia occurs as the result of
    a. repeated small strokes
    b. repeated viral infections
    c. repeated small heart attacks
    d. multiple bacteriological infections

14. Pick's disease is caused by the presence of Pick's bodies in ____.
    a. the basal ganglia
    b. muscle cells
    c. nerve cells
    d. the prefrontal cortex

15. Parkinson's disease is caused by the destruction of ____ in the ____ of the brain.
    a. cells, basal ganglia
    b. cells, cerebral cortex
    c. neurotransmitter, basal ganglia
    d. neurotransmitter, cerebellum

16. Huntington's disease produces all but one of the following symptoms. Which symptom is not produced by Huntington's disease?
    a. jerky movement
    b. unstable mood
    c. personality change
    d. memory loss

17. Approximately, ____% of the children of a person who has Huntington's disease will also contract the disease.
    a. 100
    b. 50
    c. 10
    d. 1

18. What is the general term used to describe any infection of the brain?
    a. AIDS dementia complex
    b. general paresis
    c. encephalitis
    d. meningitis

19. Which type of brain trauma involve "bruising" the brain by a sharp blow?
    a. concussion
    b. contusion
    c. laceration
    d. melioration

20. The leakage of blood onto the brain producing brain damage is called a
    a. cerebral hemorrhage
    b. cerebral thrombosis
    c. cerebral embolism
    d. cerebral occlusion

21. Brain tumors can produce which of the following symptoms?
    a. loss of memory and disorientation
    b. impaired motor coordination and seizures
    c. personality changes and hallucinations
    d. all of the above can be produced by brain tumors

22. Thiamine deficiency is the cause of ____.
    a. beriberi
    b. pellagra
    c. hypothyroidism
    d. Addison's disease

23. Abnormally low level of thyroxin will produce ____ a disorder characterized by stunted growth and mental retardation.
    a. Addison's disease
    b. Cushing's syndrome
    c. cretinism
    d. hyperthyroidism

24. According to your text, persons with epilepsy have been humiliated ____ than persons suffering from other diseases.
    a. about the same
    b. a lot less
    c. a little more
    d. a lot more

25. Persons with ____ epilepsy retain control of their motor functions but lose contact with reality.
    a. tonic-clonic
    b. symptomatic
    c. focal
    d. temporal lobe

26. Which of the following statements is true?
    a. Having a seizure is a sure diagnostic sign that one has epilepsy.
    b. Epilepsy produces profound personality disturbances.
    c. Idiopathic epilepsy is a genetic disorder.
    d. Most epileptics do not require custodial care.

27. Which pair of the following medications is typically used to control the occurrence of seizures in epileptics?
    a. Dilantin and Ritalin
    b. Dilantin and phenobarbital
    c. phenobarbital and benzodiazapene
    d. L-dopa and phenobarbital

TERMS AND CONCEPTS

Lesson 1
agnosia (456)
organic mental disorders (457)
organic mental syndromes (458)

Lesson 2
alcohol amnestic disorder (461)
amnestic syndrome (460)
ataxia (461)
delirium (459)
delirium tremens (459)
Korsakoff's syndrome (461)

Lesson 3
Alzheimer's disease (464)
aphasia (469)
dementias (464)
Global Deterioration Scale or GDS (466)
multi-infarct dementia or MID (469)
Pick's Disease (469)
presenile demential (464)
senile dementia (464)

Lesson 4
basal ganglia (470)
Huntington's disease (471)
Parkinson's disease (470)

Lesson 5
AIDS dementia complex (473)
brain tumors (475)
cerebral hemorrhage (475)
cerebrovascular disorder (474)
concussion (473)
contusion (474)
encephalitis (472)
general paresis (472)
laceration (474)
meningitis (472)
neurosyphilis (472)
stroke (474)

Lesson 6
Addison's disease (476)
beriberi (475)
cretinism (476)
Cushing's syndrome (476)
hyperthyroidism (476)
hypothyroidism (476)
pellagra (475)
thyroxin (476)

Lesson 7
acquired epilepsy (477)
epilepsy (476)
grand mal seizure (477)
idiopathic epilepsy (477)
petit mal epilepsy (478)
tonic-clonic epilepsy (477)

TYING THINGS TOGETHER

1. After reviewing the symptoms of Alzheimer's disease, make a list of every day chores which an Alzheimer's victim would probably be incapable of doing.

2. An expression from the 1960s was "you are what you eat." Explain how this expression is true with respect to abnormal behavior.

ANSWERS

Lesson 1
1 a
2 b
3 c

Lesson 2
1 f
2 d
3 c
4 e
5 b
6 a

Lesson 3
1 h
2 g
3 a
4 b
5 f
6 e
7 d
8 c

Lesson 4
1 a
2 b
3 c

Lesson 5
1 l
2 f
3 g
4 b
5 d
6 e
7 i
8 k
9 c
10 j
11 h
12 a

Lesson 6
1 a
2 g
3 e
4 b
5 d
6 c
7 h
8 f

Lesson 7
1 c
2 a
3 f
4 d
5 e
6 b

True-False answers

1 T
2 F
3 F
4 T
5 T
6 F
7 F
8 F
9 F
10 T
11 T
12 T
13 T
14 T
15 F
16 T
17 F
18 T
19 T
20 T
21 F
22 T
23 T
24 T
25 F
26 F
27 T

Multiple-Choice answers

1 a
2 d
3 a
4 b
5 c
6 a
7 b
8 c
9 d
10 c
11 a
12 c
13 a
14 c
15 a
16 d
17 b
18 c
19 b
20 a
21 d
22 a
23 c
24 d
25 d
26 d
27 b

14 Developmental Disorders

OVERVIEW

As you should already realize, DSM-III-R and your text typically group disorders based upon the similarity of behavioral symptoms. This chapter is one of the exceptions. The developmental disorders are **not** grouped together because of symptom similarity. In fact, the characteristic behaviors of different developmental disorder are highly dissimilar. The developmental disorders are grouped together for two reasons, the age of onset of these disorders and the need to take age, sex, family, culture, and developmental level into account in making a diagnosis of these disorders. The developmental disorders are disorders of childhood and adolescence, which may or may not persist into adulthood. A behavior or behaviors which may cause one child to be diagnosed as suffering from a developmental disorder may **not** cause another child to be diagnosed because of differences in age, sex, family background, cultural background, or developmental level.

Your chapter begins with a brief discussion of the unique difficulties in diagnosing developmental disorders. That is, the problem of taking into account age, sex, family and cultural background, and developmental level in assessing the abnormality or normality of a behavior or behaviors. The chapter continues with a discussion of general risk factors for the disorders of childhood and adolescence. Then, the analysis of the major disorders of childhood and adolescence begins.

There are eight major disorders discussed in your text. They are autism, mental retardation, learning disabilities, disruptive behavior, anxiety disorders, depression, eating disorders, and elimination disorders. For each disorder, you will need to know four things: the characteristics or definition of the disorder; the risk factor and causes for the disorder; theories for the disorder; and treatments for the disorder. As you have done in the past, making a chart in your notebook will help you to organize and remember this information.

We've organized this chapter into five lessons. We'll give you more information about how to learn about the eight major disorders of childhood and adolescence in the introduction to each lesson.

CHAPTER OUTLINE, LESSONS & LEARNING OBJECTIVES

Lesson 1. Determining abnormality, risk factors, & autism. (483-491)

1. Discuss the difficulties in determining what is normal and abnormal in childhood and adolescence.

RISK FACTORS FOR DISORDERS OF CHILDHOOD AND ADOLESCENCE. (484-485)

BIO - Gender (Boys ↑ risk) Prenatal factors, genetics, illness in childhood
PSYCHSOCIAL - instability + family conflict, social acceptance, neglect, abuse,

2. Discuss the risk factors for disorders of childhood and adolescence.

AUTISM. (485-491)

3. Discuss the theories of autism. *affect cognitive, social, + emotional - Psych -*
4. Describe the difference between autism and childhood schizophrenia. *→ d/n show language + intellectu deficiencies, d/n become attached.*
5. Discuss the treatment of autism. *psychotherapy, play therapy, + placement of residential facilities*

Lesson 2. Cognitive abnormalities and deficits. (491-501)

MENTAL RETARDATION. (491-497)

6. Describe the assessment of mental retardation. *observation + testing of intelligence of functioning*
7. Identify and define the levels of mental retardation and discuss the capacities and deficits associated with each level. *Mild - 80-70 - almost self-sufficient Moderate - 35-49 - simple tasks Severe - 20-34 - daily routines Profound - < 20 Chromosomal - Down Syndrome - round face, flat nose, sloped eyes, square hands, protruding tongue Recessive Gene - phenylketonuria (P c/n met phenylalanin Tay-Sachs - degene nervous system*
8. Discuss the causes of mental retardation.
9. Describe the different methods for detecting genetic defects.
10. Describe intervention approaches to mental retardation.
11. Describe the savant syndrome. *most male, outstanding memories, autistic + / or retarded sharp mental skills.*

LEARNING DISABILITIES. (497-501) *dyslexia,*

12. Identify and define the different types of learning disabilities.
13. Discuss the theories of learning disabilities. *Cognitive - how organize thoughts Linguistic - child's language deficiencies*
14. Discuss approaches to remediating learning disabilities. *Medical - biologically based deficiencies Neuropsycho - underlying deficits in proc. info (cerebral cortex)*
Psychoed - goes on strengths + weaknesses, Behav - hierarchy of basic skills

Lesson 3. Behavioral abnormalities and deficits. (502-506)

DISRUPTIVE BEHAVIOR. (502-506)

15. Discuss the theories of attention-deficit hyperactivity disorder (ADHD)
16. Describe the treatments for ADHD and their effectiveness.
17. Discuss the theory and treatment of conduct disorders.

Lesson 4. Affective abnormalities and deficits. (506-513)

ANXIETY DISORDERS OF CHILDHOOD. (506-509)

18. Describe the diagnosis and treatment of the anxiety disorders of childhood.

DEPRESSION IN CHILDHOOD AND ADOLESCENCE. (509-513)

19. Describe the features of depression in childhood and adolescence and its treatment.
20. Discuss the risk factors for suicide in adolescence.

Lesson 5. Abnormal eating and elimination. (513-521)
EATING DISORDERS. (513-520)
21. Describe anorexia nervosa and bulimia nervosa.
22. Discuss the theories of anorexia nervosa and bulimia nervosa.
23. Describe the treatment of anorexia nervosa and bulimia nervosa.
ELIMINATION DISORDERS. (520-521)
24. Discuss the theories of functional enuresis and functional encopresis.
25. Describe the treatment of functional enuresis and functional encopresis.

Mastering Lesson 1. Determine abnormality, risk factors, & autism. (483-491)

This first lesson has three parts. The first two parts cover general background information for all of the developmental disorders. We cannot emphasize enough the importance of remembering that the diagnosis of developmental disorders requires one to take the contextual factors of age, sex, family background, cultural background, and developmental level into account. As your learn the diagnostic criteria for each of the eight major types of developmental disorders covered in your text, you should be able to indicate how changing any of these contextual factors could change a diagnosis. Second, there are a number of risk factors associated with all developmental disorders. Your text groups these as either biological or psychosocial risk factors. You will need to understand the general and disorder specific effects of these two groups of risk factors.

The first lesson ends with a discussion of the first of eight developmental disorders, autism. You will need to learn the following about autism. You need to know the basic diagnostic signs of autism which are summarized in Table 14.1 in your text and how autism differs from childhood schizophrenia. Your text examines the causes, risk factors, and theories for autism in two sections labeled "Psychological Perspectives" and "Biological Perspectives." For some developmental disorders, there is general agreement among psychologists and psychiatrists of different theoretical orientations about certain facts, which can be called causes and risk factors. In the case of autism, this general agreement does not exist. Therefore, causes and risk factors cannot be discussed separately from theoretical perspectives. Obviously, this makes your job in learning this stuff more difficult.

The first lesson ends with a discussion of available treatments for autism. Your text will indicate that behaviorally based treatments are generally the most effective but only with a limited range of behaviors. You will need to know what those behaviors are. Unfortunately, the long term prognosis for autistic children is not good.

Match the following terms and concepts with the correct definition or description or explanation.

1. _E_ autism
2. _B_ Axis I disorders
3. _G_ Axis II disorder
4. _H_ Bruno Bettleheim
5. _D_ childhood schizophrenia
6. _F_ echolalia
7. _C_ I. Ovar Lovaas
8. _A_ pervasive developmental disorder

a. abnormalities of cognitive, social, and emotional development
b. anxiety, eating, and elimination disorders
c. behavior modification through operant conditioning
d. confusion, disorientation, incoherent speech, and hallucinations
e. deficits in social interaction, communication, and activity
f. high-pitched monotonic repetition of another person's words
g. mental retardation, autism, and learning disabilities
h. psychodynamically oriented play therapy

175

Mastering Lesson 2. Cognitive abnormalities and deficits. (491-501)

Lesson 2 covers two disorders both of which are characterized by cognitive deficits, mental retardation and learning disabilities. In the case of mental retardation, the cognitive deficit is global; that is, the individual shows impaired general intelligence. In the case of learning disabilities, a person, with otherwise normal intelligence, has a specific impairment. For example, in the case of dyslexia, the person has difficulty reading even though they may completely understand the same information if it is read to them. Remember, you will need to know the characteristics or definition of the two disorders, the risk factor and causes for the two disorders, theories for the two disorders, and treatments for the disorders.

Two additional issues related to mental retardation are discussed in your text and covered in this lesson. Since genetic defect is a known cause of mental retardation, methods for detecting genetic defects are discussed. Finally, some individuals who are otherwise retarded can show above normal cognitive abilities. The so-called "savant syndrome" has intrigued and mystified since its discovery. We expect that you will feel the same way. You will also need to understand these two issues

Match the following terms and concepts with the correct definition or description or explanation.

1. E	academic skills disorders	a.	autistic or retarded persons with one exceptional mental ability
2. D	cultural-familial retardation	b.	fatal degenerative disease of the central nervous system
3. Q	Down syndrome	c.	impaired reading ability in a normally intelligent person
4. C	dyslexia	d.	impoverished social environment producing mental retardation
5. J	fetal alcohol syndrome	e.	inadequate arithmetic, writing, and reading skills
6. K	IQ score 20-34	f.	inadequate articulation, speaking, and listening skills
7. J	IQ score 35-49	g.	inadequate development of a specific intellectual skill
8. R	IQ score 50-70	h.	IQ of 70 or below, impaired adaptive functioning, before age 18
9. O	IQ score below 20	i.	marked delay in motor development and no communication skills
10. F	language and speech disorders	j.	mental retardation due to alcohol abuse by mothers
11. G	learning disability	k.	mild mental retardation
12. H	mental retardation	l.	moderate mental retardation
13. M	mild mental retardation	m.	not noticed as retarded by a casual observer
14. N	moderate mental retardation	n.	noticeable delay in motor development and responds to training
15. S	phenylketonuria (PKU)	o.	profound mental retardation
16. P	profound mental retardation	p.	requires nursing care and has minimal sensorimotor functions
17. A	savant syndrome	q.	round face, broad flat nose, small hands, and mentally retarded
18. I	severe mental retardation	r.	severe mental retardation
19. B	Tay-Sachs disease	s.	unable to metabolize an amino acid

176

Mastering Lesson 3. Behavioral abnormalities and deficits. 502-506)

Lesson 3 covers disruptive behavior of childhood and adolescence. Your text examines two major disruptive behavior disorders, attention-deficit hyperactivity disorder (ADHD) and conduct disorder. As in the past, your task is to learn the characteristics or definition for these disorders; the risk factor and causes for these disorders; theories for the disorders; and treatments for the disorders. You'll need to pay particular attention to Table 14.5 of your text.

Match the following terms and concepts with the correct definition or description or explanation.

1. _C_ attention-deficit hyperactivity disorder
2. _D_ conduct disorder
3. _B_ disruptive behavior disorders
4. _A_ Ritalin

a.   a stimulant drug used to treat hyperactive children
b.   behavior which is socially disruptive and upsetting to others
c.   inappropriate impulsivity, inattention, and hyperactivity
d.   intentional antisocial behavior

Mastering Lesson 4. Affective abnormalities and deficits. (506-513)

Lessons 1 and 2 covered cognitive abnormalities in childhood and adolescence. Lesson 3 covered behavioral abnormalities. In the triad of affect, behavior, and cognition, this leaves affect, another word for emotion. Lesson 4 covers affective abnormalities, emotional disorders, in childhood and adolescence. Your text discusses two classes of emotional disorders, anxiety disorders of childhood and depression in childhood and adolescence.

Your text discusses three anxiety disorders of childhood: separation anxiety disorder, avoidant disorder, and overanxious disorder. For each of these three disorders and depression, you will need to know the diagnostic characteristics, the risk factors and causes, theories of their occurrence, and treatment for them. If you are making a table or matrix, the table will have sixteen cells, four disorders with four cells for each. In a manner similar to the discussion of depression and suicide in adults, your text examines the relationship of depression to suicide in children and adolescents. Therefore, you will need to know the risk factors for suicide in adolescence and how to prevent suicide in adolescence.

Match the following terms and concepts with the correct definition or description or explanation.

1. _D_ avoidant disorder
2. _B_ depression of childhood and adolescence
3. _A_ overanxious disorder
4. _C_ separation anxiety disorder

a.   a generalized fear or anxiety about past, present, and future events
b.   broad negative expectancies and catastrophizing
c.   excessive and inappropriate fear of separation from a care-giver
d.   excessive fear of contact with strangers including other children

177

Mastering Lesson 5. Abnormal eating and elimination. (513-521)

Even planaria (single celled organisms) eat and eliminate. Therefore, one might expect that such "simple" behaviors might be immune to disruption. Unfortunately, that's not the case. There are four disorders covered in the last two sections of your text, "Elimination Disorders" and "Eating Disorders." Make a table in your notebook summarizing the characteristics and definitions of anorexia nervosa, bulimia nervosa, functional enuresis, and functional encopresis. Tables 14.6 and 14.7 of your text summarize the diagnostic criteria for anorexia and bulimia. You'll have to dig out criteria for enuresis and encopresis from the narrative in you text. Fill out your table with the risk factors and causes for these four disorders, theories, and treatments.

Match the following terms and concepts with the correct definition or description or explanation.

1. _C_ anorexia nervosa
2. _E_ bulimia nervosa
3. _B_ functional encopresis
4. _A_ functional enuresis
5. _D_ systems perspective

a. a failure to control one's bladder past the age of 5
b. a failure to control one's bowels past the age of 4
c. an intense fear of overweight combined with abnormally low weight
d. families are systems which attempt to minimize conflict and change
e. recurrent pattern of excessive eating followed by purging

PRACTICE EXAM

Exam 1. (true-false)

Indicate whether each of the following statements is **True** or **False**. Question numbers correspond to learning objectives from which the questions were drawn.

1. _T_ Age is a critical factor in the diagnosis of childhood and adolescent disorders.
2. _F_ Stress in childhood is rare and therefore is not a risk factor for childhood disorders.
3. _F_ There is clear evidence that emotional detachment and rejection by parents causes autism.
4. _F_ Childhood schizophrenia is autism developed earlier in life.
5. _F_ ~~_T_~~ Autistic children will stop engaging in self-mutilation if it produces an external painful stimulus.
6. _F_ If a person has an IQ of 65, then we know that they are retarded.
7. _F_ As adults, the mentally retarded need constant supervision.
8. _T_ German measles, syphilis, and herpes in a mother increases the risk of mental retardation in her children.
9. _T_ Down syndrome is detectable through a blood test of a pregnant women.
10. _T_ The mentally retarded have the legal right to live in the least restrictive environment possible.
11. _F_ ~~_T_~~ Savants are more likely to be retarded than autistic.
12. _T_ Dyslexia is the inability to read fluently.
13. _T_ Learning disabilities tend to run in families.
14. _T_ The psychoeducational model of treatment for learning disabilities does not attempt to correct deficiencies.
15. _F_ Mothers who use alcohol are more likely to have children with ADHD than mothers who do not.

178

16. _T_ The most common treatment for ADHD is drug therapy.
17. _T_ Psychotherapy is generally ineffective in treating conduct disorders in children.
18. _F_ The developmentally normal fear of strangers disappears by age 1 year.
19. _T_ Children who suffer from depression may be unaware of it.
20. _T_ The suicide rate for adolescents has tripled in the last 30 years.
21. _T_ Anorexia nervosa is more likely to occur in girls than boys.
22. _T_ Families of anorexics and bulemics show greater disfunction than the families of "normal" adolescents.
23. _T_ Anorexics who return to "normal" weight following therapy often believe that they are overweight.
24. _T_ MZ twins show higher concordance for functional enuresis than DZ twins.
25. _F_ Functional enuresis if left untreated will get worse.

Exam 2 (multiple-choice)

Select the single, best answer for each question. Question numbers correspond to learning objectives from which the questions were drawn.

1. Disorders of childhood and adolescence which are classified on Axis II of DSM-III-R
   a. persist into adulthood
   b. occur only in adolescence
   c. occur only in childhood
   d. are childhood anxiety disorders

2. Disorders of anxiety and depression in childhood are more likely to be found in ____; in adolescence, they are more likely to be found in ____.
   a. boys; boys
   b. boys; girls
   c. girls; boys
   d. girls; girls

3. Studies of the genetics of autism in MZ twins find
   a. 100% concordance proving that defective genes produce autism
   b. 100% concordance proving that the environment must play some role
   c. well less than 100% concordance proving that the environment must play some role
   d. well less than 100% concordance proving nothing about the role of the environment

4. In DSM-III-R, childhood schizophrenia
   a. is diagnosed by markedly different symptoms than adult schizophrenia
   b. is diagnosed by the presence of hallucinations at 20 months
   c. was replaced by the name autistic disorder for the same symptoms
   d. is not a diagnostic classification

5. Research indicates that ____ treatment is effective in improving the IQ scores of autistic children.
   a. psychodynamic
   b. humanist-existential
   c. behavioral
   d. drug

6. For an individual to be diagnosed as mentally retarded, they must meet three of the following diagnostic criteria. Which of the following is <u>not</u> one of the criteria for mental retardation?
   a. IQ of 70 or below
   b. impaired adaptive behavior
   c. evidence of disorder before age 18
   d. a history of violent behavior

7. As an adult, a person can perform simple tasks under sheltered conditions but is incapable of self-maintenance. This person shows _____ mental retardation.
   a. mild
   b. moderate
   c. severe
   d. profound

8. You place an infant on a diet low in the protein phenylalanine to prevent mental retardation due to
   a. Down syndrome
   b. PKU syndrome
   c. fetal alcohol syndrome
   d. cultural-familial retardation

9. Amniocentesis
   a. is a genetic defect causing blindness
   b. is a blood disease of pregnant women
   c. involves drawing fluid from the uterus
   d. is done 9-12 weeks after conception

10. A person with which level of retardation is most likely to benefit from being "mainstreamed" in school?
    a. profound
    b. severe
    c. moderate
    d. mild

11. The special skills demonstrated by savants are usually associated with which brain functions?
    a. right hemisphere functions
    b. left hemisphere functions
    c. hypothalamic functions
    d. occipital cortex functions

12. Which of the following is an example of a language and speech disorder in DSM-III-R?
    a. developmental arithmetic disorder
    b. developmental expressive writing disorder
    c. developmental reading disorder
    d. developmental articulation disorder

180

13. Current research and theory of learning disabilities is focused on cognitive-perceptual problems which result from
    a. underlying neurological problems
    b. Downs syndrome
    c. id-superego conflicts
    d. ideo-motor conflict syndrome

14. Treatment based upon which model has produced impressive improvements in the skills of children with learning disabilities?
    a. psychoeducational
    b. medical
    c. neuropsychological
    d. behavioral

15. The nervous systems of boys develop ____ than girls and boys are ____ likely than girls to develop attention-deficit hyperactivity disorder.
    a. slower; more
    b. slower; less
    c. faster; less
    d. faster; more

16. Treating children with ADHD with stimulant drugs
    a. elicits aggressive behavior
    b. reduces disruptive classroom activity
    c. disrupts voluntary motor activity
    d. improves general academic achievement

17. Aggressive children with conduct disorders assume that other persons are trying to
    a. harm them, when the other person is
    b. harm them, when the other person is not
    c. help them, when the other person is
    d. help them, when the other person is not

18. When a child shows excessive and developmentally inappropriate fear of being removed from her or his mother, the child may suffer from what disorder?
    a. separation anxiety disorder
    b. avoidant disorder
    c. overanxious disorder
    d. oppositional defiant disorder

19. Which of the following is not one of the symptoms of childhood depression?
    a. broad negative expectations for the future
    b. underestimating the consequences of negative events
    c. incorrectly assuming responsibility for negative events
    d. selectively attending to negative aspects of events

20. Which of the following would increase the likelihood of an adolescent committing suicide?
    a. if they are a girl instead of a boy
    b. if they come from the city instead of the country
    c. if they are older instead of younger
    d. if they know someone who has committed suicide

21. One in ___ female adolescents meets the DSM-III-R diagnostic criteria for anorexia nervosa.
    a. 100
    b. 1,000
    c. 100,000
    d. 1,000,000

22. In comparison with normal families, families of anorexics and bulemics show more
    a. cohesion
    b. emotional expression
    c. autonomy training
    d. conflict

23. Having a bulemic eat forbidden foods and then preventing them from purging themselves
    a. is an effective treatment
    b. produces psychotic responses
    c. is an untested therapy
    d. causes them to become anorexic

24. Which theoretical perspective suggests that functional enuresis is the result of attempting to toilet train too early?
    a. behavioral
    b. genetic
    c. humanist-existential
    d. psychodynamic

25. Mowrer's bell-and-pad treatment for functional enuresis creates a waking response as a conditioned response to the conditioned stimulus of
    a. the ringing bell
    b. bladder tension
    c. the wet pad or bed
    d. sleeping

TERMS AND CONCEPTS

Lesson 1
autism (486)
Axis I disorders (484)
Axis II disorder (484)
Bruno Bettleheim (488)
childhood schizophrenia (490)
echolalia (486)
I. Ovar Lovaas (488)
pervasive developmental disorder (486)

Lesson 2
academic skills disorders (497)
cultural-familial retardation (495)
Down syndrome (492)
dyslexia (497)
fetal alcohol syndrome (495)
IQ score 20-34 (491)
IQ score 35-49 (491)
IQ score 50-70 (491)
IQ score below 20 (491)
language and speech disorders (499)
learning disability (497)
mental retardation (491)
mild mental retardation (492)
moderate mental retardation (492)
phenylketonuria (PKU) (494)
profound mental retardation (492)
savant syndrome (498)
severe mental retardation (492)
Tay-Sachs disease (494)

Lesson 3
attention-deficit hyperactivity disorder (502)
conduct disorder (505)
disruptive behavior disorders (502)
Ritalin (503)

Lesson 4
avoidant disorder (509)
depression of childhood and adolescence (510)
overanxious disorder (509)
separation anxiety disorder (508)

Lesson 5
anorexia nervosa (514)
bulimia nervosa (515)
functional encopresis (521)
functional enuresis (520)
systems perspective (518)

TYING THINGS TOGETHER

1. Make a list of the last five jobs you've had. If you haven't had five paying jobs count jobs around the house. For each job indicate the key skills required to do the job. After reviewing the material in your text, indicate which of these jobs could be done by a moderately and mildly retarded person. Justify you answer. *This can prove to be a very humbling experience. RAH paid for his first three years of college (which took four years to complete) doing jobs which could have been done by a mildly retarded person. Also keep in mind, that retarded workers usually have lower absenteeism rates than non-retarded workers.*

2. Section 504 of the Rehabilitation Act of 1972 requires colleges and universities to accommodate the needs of students with learning disabilities. Find the Section 504 Coordinator on your campus and ask her or him to provide you with five examples of the ways in which your school has accommodated students with learning disabilities.

3. With a developmental disorder, the age of onset of the disorder, sex, family, culture, and developmental level need to be taken into account in making a diagnosis of a disorder. Show how this would be true for a diagnosis of depression.

ANSWERS

Lesson 1
1 e
2 b
3 g
4 h
5 d
6 f
7 c
8 a

Lesson 2
1 e
2 d
3 q
4 c
5 j
6 k
7 i
8 r
9 o
10 f
11 g
12 h
13 m
14 n
15 s
16 p
17 a
18 i
19 b

Lesson 3
1 c
2 d
3 b
4 a

Lesson 4
1 d
2 b
3 a
4 c

Lesson 5
1 c
2 e
3 b
4 a
5 d

T r u e - F a l s e answers

1 T
2 F
3 F
4 F
5 T
6 F
7 F
8 T
9 T
10 T
11 T
12 T
13 T
14 T
15 T
16 T
17 T
18 F
19 T
20 T
21 T
22 T
23 T
24 T
25 F

Multiple-Choice answers

1 a
2 b
3 c
4 d
5 c
6 d
7 b
8 b
9 c
10 d
11 a
12 d
13 a
14 d
15 a
16 b
17 b
18 a
19 b
20 d
21 a
22 d
23 a
24 a
25 b

15 Methods of Therapy and Treatment

OVERVIEW

Chapter 15 "Methods of Therapy and Treatment" examines five different types of therapy. The five types are psychodynamic therapies, humanist-existential therapies, cognitive therapies, behavior therapy, and biological therapies. Each of these therapies is based upon a different perspective of abnormal behavior. These perspectives were examined in detail in Chapter 2 "Theoretical Perspectives." Therefore, Chapter 2 is a good place to start in preparing to understand the material of Chapter 15. A thorough understanding of the material of Chapter 2 will make understanding Chapter 15 considerable easier. Before you read Chapter 15, you might reread the summary of Chapter 2, pages 74-77 of your text, to refresh your memory.

Chapter 15 opens by developing a definition of what psychotherapy is. The chapter continues by describing the four major types of psychologically based psychotherapy in separate sections. Those sections are "Psychodynamic Therapies,""Humanist-Existential Therapies,""Cognitive Therapies," and "Behavior Therapy." We call these therapies psychological because they look for causes and treatment for abnormal behavior in the feelings, behavior, and thoughts of the individual instead of their biology. (Biologically based therapies are covered later.) Each section follows a similar format as indicated by the learning objective for these four sections. The section begins with a brief review of the philosophy and goals for that psychotherapy. The section continues with a straightforward description of psychotherapeutic methods for that therapy.

Traditionally, psychotherapy has been done on individuals, however, there are alternative methods. Therefore, after examining the four major psychological psychotherapies, your chapter examines two alternative methods of providing therapy, "Group Therapy" and "Family Therapy." The analysis of psychological psychotherapies ends with the consideration of an extremely controversial topic, which your text does not and could not cover in detail. The topic is the effectiveness of psychotherapy. Research on this subject is not clear cut. There is no indisputable evidence that psychotherapy is effective.

The section ends with two sections on medical psychotherapy. The first section examines biological therapies, which include chemotherapy, electroconvulsive therapy, and psychosurgery. All of these medical psychotherapies are also controversial. The last section of the chapter examines the changing role of the state mental hospital, which has traditionally used medical psychotherapeutic techniques, primarily chemotherapy.

CHAPTER OUTLINE, LESSONS & LEARNING OBJECTIVES

Lesson 1. Psychoanalysis: gaining insight into unconscious conflicts. (526-530)
PSYCHOTHERAPY (526-527)
1. Define psychotherapy. *systematic interaction btwn a client + therapist that incorporates psych principles + help being Δ in behavior, thoughts, feeling to help client overcome abnorm behav*
PSYCHODYNAMIC THERAPIES (527-530)
2. Describe the goals and methods of traditional psychoanalysis.
3. Compare and contrast traditional psychoanalysis with modern psychodynamic approaches.
T → use free assoc, + dream analysis, + transference
M → psychoanalytic psychotherapy, focus on current relationships

Lesson 2. Humanist-existential therapies: gaining insight into meaning. (530-533)
HUMANIST-EXISTENTIAL THERAPIES (530-533) *focus on subjective, conscious experiences*
4. Describe the philosophies and goals of humanistic-existential therapies.
5. Describe person-centered, gestalt, and existential therapies.
P-C - non-directive, Rogers, more aware + accepting of their true selves, uncon. + regard, empathetic understanding, Genuin Congr
G - Perls, direct, confrontational, hostile, blend conflicting parts of personality. Ex - more aware of conscious experiences, + make p choices to give life meaning + fulfil Frankl

Lesson 3. Cognitive therapies: changing people's thoughts. (533-535)
COGNITIVE THERAPIES (533-535)
6. Describe the philosophies and goals of cognitive therapies.
7. Compare and contrast the methods of rational-emotive therapy with Beck's cognitive therapy. *RET - directive, pinpoint irrational beliefs, showing how beliefs lead to personal misery, challenging their valid + finding workable alternatives, Ellis*
COG - encourage to recognize how errors in thinking affect mood, + impair behavior, cog-behavioral therapy

Lesson 4. Behavior therapy: changing people's behavior. (535-540)
BEHAVIOR THERAPY (535-540) *SD - reduce fear + phobia by combining muscle relaxation w/ imaginal exposures to s thru a sequence*
GE - real life AC - connects fear w/ problem behaviors
8. Describe the philosophies and goals of behavior therapy. *OC - reinforcement principles*
9. Describe systematic desensitization, gradual exposure, aversive conditioning, operant conditioning, social skills training, and methods for fostering self-control. *SST - counter social anxiet, more effective social s*
ECLECTICISM IN PSYCHOTHERAPY (540) *SC - changing antecedents (A's) that trigger prob. behavio + reinforcement consequences that follow (C's)*
10. Explain what is meant by eclecticism in psychotherapy.
Incorporate principles + techniques from dif. therapeutic orientations

Lesson 5. Alternative methods for delivering therapy. (540-543)
GROUP THERAPY (540-542) *gter access to limited therapist resources, deal more effectively wi ↑ info + experience to draw on, source of hope people.*
11. Describe the advantages of group therapy. *less costly, grp support, probs not unique,*
12. Describe psychodrama and encounter groups. *P → Moreno, role-play*
E - ↑ self awareness, Relations w/ others in grp.
FAMILY THERAPY (542-543)
13. Describe family therapy approaches to treating the family unit.

Lesson 6. Evaluating the effectiveness of psychotherapy. (543-547)
EVALUATING THE EFFECTIVENESS OF PSYCHOTHERAPY (543-547)
14. Summarize the research issues in evaluating the effectiveness of psychotherapy.
15. Describe the technique of meta-analysis.
16. Summarize the findings of research into the effectiveness of psychotherapy.
Client, Therapist + Treatment factors

Lesson 7. Biological and medical therapies. (547-558)
BIOLOGICAL THERAPIES (547-552)
   17. Describe the uses and abuses of chemotherapy.
   18. Describe electroconvulsive therapy and explain why it is controversial.
   19. Describe the prefrontal lobotomy and explain why it is controversial.
HOSPITALIZATION AND COMMUNITY-BASED CARE (552-558)
   20. Describe the contemporary roles for hospitalization and for community mental health centers.
   21. Identify and describe the problems of deinstitutionalization.

Mastering Lesson 1. Psychoanalysis: gaining insight into unconscious conflicts. (526-530)

This first lessons covers three topics. The first two topics are brief and clear, what psychotherapy is and who does it. For the first, you need to learn a relatively straight forward definition of psychotherapy. There are four defining characteristics of psychotherapy. Those characteristics are described on page 526 of your text. For the second, you need to become familiar with three different types of helping professionals.

The third topic of this lesson is psychoanalysis, the psychotherapy based upon the psychoanalytic theory of Sigmund Freud. As you should remember from Chapter 2, psychoanalytic theory is complex. You had to learn a large number of concepts and processes. Likewise, you will need to do the same thing to begin to understand psychoanalysis, which can be adequately described only through a large number of concepts and processes. Your chapter's brief introduction to psychanalysis describes some of the more important concepts and processes. We have attempted to include all of those concepts and processes in the lesson exam below.

Match the following terms and concepts with the correct definition or description or explanation.

1. I clinical psychologist
2. D countertransference
3. F dream analysis
4. K ego analysis
5. R free association
6. P insight
7. Q latent content
8. M manifest content
9. J modern psychodynamic approaches
10. L object-relations therapy
11. H psychiatric social worker
12. G psychiatrist
13. C psychoanalysis
14. A psychotherapy
15. B resistance
16. S traditional psychoanalysis
17. E transference
18. O transference neurosis
19. N transference relationship

a. a systematic interaction using psychological principles to change a client's abnormal behavior

b. an unwillingness or inability to recall or discuss ego threatening material

c. the therapy which attempts to gain insight into unconscious conflicts and resolve them

d. displacement of feelings onto a client by a therapist

e. displacement of feelings toward a parent onto one's therapist

f. examination of manifest and latent content

g. MD or DO with a residency in diagnosis and treatment

h. MSW trained to utilize social support services and agencies

i. PhD trained in the assessment, diagnosis, and treatment

j. psychoanalysis emphasizing a client's current relationships

k. psychoanalysis emphasizing the importance of the ego

l. psychoanalysis emphasizing the separation of personal from introjected feelings

m. the content of a dream that a dreamer experiences

n. the development of a transference neurosis with one's therapist

o. the reenactment of childhood parental conflicts with one's therapist

p. the relatively sudden understanding of deep-seated conflicts and feelings

q. the unconscious material symbolized by dream content

r. therapeutic technique of uttering thoughts as they enter consciousness

s. therapy originated by Sigmund Freud

Mastering Lesson 2. Humanist-existential therapies: gaining insight into meaning. (530-533)

This lesson examines three therapies. They are person-centered therapy, Gestalt therapy, and logotherapy. The terms used to describe these therapies and the methods employed to produce change may be different but these therapies share a similar philosophy. The humanist-existential therapies share the belief that the subjective, conscious experience of a client should be the focus of therapy. In addition, all of these therapies assume that abnormal behavior reflects a lack of meaning and coherence to the client's life.

You will need to learn names of the individual's identified with each of the three therapies. You will need to learn how these therapies are conducted, that is, the techniques employed by the therapy. Since, there are specific names or terms by which those techniques are identified, you will need to know those terms.

Match the following terms and concepts with the correct definition or description or explanation.

1. _I_ congruence
2. _J_ dialogue
3. _G_ e m p a t h e t i c understanding
4. _A_ Fritz Perls
5. _H_ genuineness
6. _D_ Gestalt therapy
7. _K_ humanistic-existential therapies
8. _E_ logotherapy
9. _L_ person-centered/client-centered therapy
10. _C_ Carl Rogers
11. _F_ unconditional positive regard
12. _B_ Victor Frankl

a. developer of Gestalt therapy
b. developer of logotherapy
c. developer of client-centered therapy
d. emphasizes a client's subjective experience in the here and now
e. emphasizes finding meaning in the lives of clients
f. in client-centered therapy, accepting clients without any evaluation of them or their behavior
g. in client-centered therapy, accurately reflecting a client's feelings
h. in client-centered therapy, the honest expression of feelings by a therapist
i. in client-centered therapy, the consistency among feelings, behavior, and thoughts
j. technique of Gestalt therapy to increase awareness of internal conflicts
k. therapy focusing on a client's subjective, conscious experience
l. therapy which is nondirective

Mastering Lesson 3. Cognitive therapies: changing people's thoughts. (533-535)

This lesson examines two therapies, which are very similar. Rational-emotive therapy and Beck's cognitive therapy share the assumption that abnormal behavior is the result of the adoption of irrational and self-defeating beliefs. Therefore, both therapies employ techniques aimed at changing those beliefs. The primary difference in these therapies is, as your text book suggests, one of "therapeutic style." Even though the difference is only stylistic, you should have a clear understanding of the difference.

You will need to learn names of the individual's identified with the two therapies. You will need to learn the techniques employed by those therapies and the specific names or terms by which those techniques are identified.

Match the following terms and concepts with the correct definition or description or explanation.

1. A Aaron Beck
2. B Albert Ellis
3. E Beck's cognitive therapy
4. C cognitive therapies
5. D rational-emotive therapy

a. developed Beck's cognitive therapy
b. developed rational-emotive therapy
c. focus on changing maladaptive thoughts into accurate ones
d. frees clients of irrational beliefs through direct confrontation
e. therapy which asks clients to engage in reality testing

Mastering Lesson 4. Behavior therapy: changing people's behavior. (535-540)

The lesson covers two sections of your text. The first one on behavior therapy is relatively long; the second on "Eclecticism In Psychotherapy" is relatively short.

The section on behavior therapy begins with a statement of the goals of behavior therapy. In contrast, to the previous three types of therapies we have encountered, behavior therapy treats the abnormal behavior of the client as the problem and focuses on changing it directly. This section continues with a discussion of the techniques of behavior therapy. You will need to know what the techniques are and the disorders for which they are used. You should be able to describe the following techniques: 1. assertiveness training, 2. aversive conditioning, 3. biofeedback training, 4. cognitive-behavior therapy, 5. covert sensitization, 6. gradual exposure, 7. modeling, 8. operant conditioning, 9. self-monitoring, 10. social skills training, 11. systematic desensitization, and 12. token-economy.

This lesson ends with a brief section indicating that practitioners, those doing psychotherapy, are becoming more eclectic in their orientation to therapy. This reflects the tendency of clinical psychology training programs to provide training in more than one therapeutic orientation. You can prove this to yourself by carefully looking at and understanding Figure 15-1 on page 539 of your text.

Match the following terms and concepts with the correct definition or description or explanation.

1. D assertiveness training
2. J aversive conditioning
3. B behavior therapy
4. M biofeedback training
5. N cognitive-behavior therapy
6. K covert sensitization
7. F eclecticism
8. H gradual exposure
9. O modeling
10. P operant conditioning
11. C self-control techniques
12. I self-monitoring
13. E social skills training
14. L symptom-substitution
15. G systematic desensitization
16. A token-economy

a. a system of applying operant conditioning principles to institutions
b. application of learning theory to change maladaptive behavior
c. assertiveness training, self-monitoring, modeling, & behavioral rehearsal
d. behavioral training to say no to unreasonable demands
e. changing the A's, B's, and C's of maladaptive behavior
f. changing therapeutic techniques for different abnormal behaviors
g. combines muscle relaxation with imagination of phobic stimuli
h. exposure to anxiety provoking stimuli while remaining relaxed
i. keeping a running diary of maladaptive behavior
j. pairing painful stimuli with unwanted responses
k. pairing painful stimuli with unwanted responses in the imagination
l. the belief that new symptoms will emerge to replace old ones
m. using bodily feedback in behavior therapy
n. using cognitive and behavioral therapeutic techniques together
o. using observational learning to treat phobias
p. using reinforcement principles to learn adaptive behaviors

Mastering Lesson 5. Alternative methods for delivering therapy. (540-543)

Psychotherapy is usually done on individuals. There are alternative methods of providing therapy. The sections "Group Therapy" and "Family Therapy" cover these methods. If you can clearly answer the questions posed by the learning objectives, you should have little trouble with this lesson.

Match the following terms and concepts with the correct definition or description or explanation.

1. B encounter groups
2. D family therapy
3. E group therapy
4. A psychodrama
5. C structural family therapy

a. conflict reenactment in group therapy
b. group therapy which seeks to foster self-awareness
c. sees abnormal behavior as belonging to the family
d. treating a family as a single unit
e. treating a group of clients with similar problems

Mastering Lesson 6. Evaluating the effectiveness of psychotherapy. (543-547)

This lesson considers this extremely controversial topic, which your text does not and could not cover in detail. Research on this subject is not clear cut. There is no indisputable evidence that psychotherapy is effective. You will need to know why. The short answer is that there are so many factors which influence psychotherapy (see Table 15.1, page 543) and so many ways to measure the effectiveness of psychotherapy (see Table 15.2, page 545). You will need to know and understand the information that these two tables summarize on this issue. You should also know by name the two major studies on effectiveness discussed in your text, Eysenck (1952) and Smith & Glass (1977).

Match the following terms and concepts with the correct definition or description or explanation.

1. _K_ client factors
2. _E_ Eysenck (1952)
3. _G_ meta-analysis
4. _A_ outcome measure: behavioral
5. _D_ outcome measure: personal growth
6. _C_ outcome measure: physiological
7. _I_ outcome measure: reports from others
8. _H_ outcome measure: self-report
9. _E_ Smith & Glass (1977)
10. _J_ therapist factors
11. _B_ treatment factors

a. direct observation of problem
b. frequency and length or treatment
c. heart rate, EEG, & GSR
d. measures of self-actualization
e. meta-analysis which found psychotherapy was effective
f. meta-analysis which found psychotherapy was ineffective
g. statistical averaging of many studies
h. symptom complaints
i. therapist reports or ratings
j. training and level of experience
k. type of problem or diagnostic category

Mastering Lesson 7. Biological and medical therapies. (547-558)

The final lesson of this chapter covers two topics, biological therapies and deinstitutionalization. The first topic requires you to understand three biologically based therapies, chemotherapy, ECT, and psychosurgery. You will learn the disorders for which each of these techniques is appropriate and that there is considerable controversy around their use. All of the biological techniques have side effects which may be more severe than the disorders they are designed to cure.

To fully understand chemotherapy you will need to know the information summarized in Table 15.3 (on page 551). DON'T PANIC when you look at this table. The table contains a lot of information, more information than can be digested and learned at one glance. In the exercises in this study guide, we have asked questions which require you to know the categories, some of the drug classes, and some of the trade names of drugs. Your instructor may want you to know more or know less. YOU SHOULD ASK YOUR INSTRUCTOR SPECIFICALLY HOW MUCH OF THE INFORMATION IN TABLE 15.3 YOU NEED TO KNOW. This lesson will be either easy or difficult depending upon that answer. In any case, this table is a handy guide to psychotropic drugs. Good luck.

The last section of the chapter covers deinstutionalization. Deinstitutionalization is a systematic program to remove patients from mental hospitals and place them in the community. This section will tell you why this was a good idea at the time and why deinstitutionalization hasn't succeeded.

Match the following terms and concepts with the correct definition or description or explanation.

1. _D_ antidepressants
2. _F_ biological psychiatry
3. _H_ chemotherapy
4. _I_ community mental health centers
5. _L_ deinstitutionalization
6. _G_ electroconvulsive therapy
7. _E_ major tranquilizers
8. _B_ MAO inhibitors
9. _C_ phenothiazines
10. _K_ prefrontal lobotomy
11. _J_ rebound anxiety
12. _A_ tricyclics

a. a class of antidepressants which includes Elavil and Sinequan
b. a class of antidepressants which includes Nardil and Marplan
c. a class of major tranquilizers which includes Thorazine and Mellaril
d. drugs used to treat depressive disorders
e. drugs used to treat hallucination, delusions, and confusion states
f. investigates biological defects that might explain abnormal behavior
g. passing electric shock through a person's head
h. prescribing drugs as treatment for abnormal behavior
i. primary function is to help discharged mental patients
j. return of even more severe anxiety following use of tranquilizers
k. severing the nerve running between the thalamus and prefrontal cortex
l. shifting mental health care from hospitals to communities

PRACTICE EXAM

Exam 1. (true-false)

Indicate whether each of the following statements is **True** or **False**. Question numbers correspond to learning objectives from which the questions were drawn.

1. _F_ Only psychiatrists can provide psychotherapy.
2. _T_ The goal of traditional psychoanalysis is to replace defensive behavior with adaptive behavior.
3. _F_ Object-relations therapy is an example of traditional psychoanalysis.
4. _F_ Humanist-existential approaches to therapy emphasize an objective appraisal of events.
5. _T_ According to Carl Rogers, therapists should unconditionally accept a client even if the therapist objects to some client behaviors.
6. _F_ Cognitive therapists like humanist-existential therapists focus on clients' deep feelings.
7. _T_ According to Albert Ellis and RET therapy, telling a client that their beliefs are wrong is helpful.
8. _T_ Behavior therapy focuses on altering maladaptive behavior without regard to deeper feelings and meaning.
9. _F_ Behavior therapy cannot help a person develop greater self-control because it focuses on behavior.
10. _F_ An eclectic psychotherapist primarily uses psychoanalysis.
11. _F_ Group therapy is a form of therapy used by psychoanalysts exclusively.
12. _F_ Sigmund Freud developed the group therapy technique psychodrama.

13. _T_ In family therapy, a person showing maladaptive behavior does not have a problem; a family does.

14. _F_ Measuring therapy outcomes is relatively easy.

15. _F_ Meta-analysis is a psychodynamic technique developed by Meta Hartmann.

16. _T_ Hans Eysenck found that two-thirds of neurotics improved without psychotherapy in two years.

17. _T_ Regular use of psychotherapeutic drugs requires increasingly higher doses to produce beneficial effects.

18. _F_ The effects of ECT on the brain are well understood.

19. _F_ An impaired ability to learn and reduced creativity are two side effects of prefrontal lobotomy.

20. _F_ The state mental hospital provides treatment for people unable to function, with the help of community mental health centers.

21. _T_ In general, deinstitutionalization has been a failure.

Exam 2 (multiple-choice)

Select the single, best answer for each question. Question numbers correspond to learning objectives from which the questions were drawn.

1. The definition of psychotherapy included all but one of the following. Which of the following is not one of defining characteristics of psychotherapy?
   - a. Psychotherapy involves the use of psychological principles, research, and theory
   - b. Psychotherapy can relieve abnormal behavior, develop problem solving skills, and promote personal growth
   - c. Psychotherapy changes behavior, thoughts, and feelings
   - d. All psychotherapy involves using the same fundamental system of interaction

2. A therapist is having trouble at home with his or her spouse. Soon, the therapist is arguing more and more with clients. This would be an example of what principle?
   - a. manifest content
   - b. resistance
   - c. transference
   - d. countertransference

3. Modern psychodynamic approaches are _____ than traditional psychoanalysis.
   - a. longer
   - b. less direct
   - c. more id focused
   - d. more ego focused

4. Humanist-existential approaches to therapy differ from psychoanalytic approaches by
   - a. emphasizing the past
   - b. trying to achieve insight
   - c. emphasizing conscious conflicts
   - d. trying to overcome congruence

196

5. If a therapist asks a client to confront opposing elements in his or her personality, the therapist is attempting to establish
   a. congruence
   b. dialogue
   c. empathetic understanding
   d. genuineness

6. According to cognitive therapists, which of the following is true?
   a. Abnormal feelings produce abnormal behavior
   b. Unconscious thoughts produce abnormal behavior
   c. Awareness of childhood thinking leads to adaptive adult behavior
   d. Maladaptive, automatic thoughts produce abnormal behavior

7. Asking a client to act inconsistently with their beliefs to check their accuracy is called
   a. behavior modification
   b. congruence checking
   c. reality testing
   d. logotherapizing

8. Which of the following is most likely to be a treatment goal of a behavior therapist dealing with a depressed person?
   a. develop a positive self image in the client
   b. gain insight into troubling, sibling conflicts
   c. increase the frequency of going to the movies
   d. uncover the childhood trauma leading to the depression

9. Which of the following behavior therapy techniques requires the client to use his or her imagination?
   a. modeling
   b. gradual exposure
   c. covert sensitization
   d. aversive conditioning

10. During the 1940s and 1950s, most psychotherapists were
    a. eclectic
    b. person-centered
    c. psychodynamic
    d. behavioral

11. Which of the following statements is _not_ true about group therapy?
    a. Group therapy is more efficient because one can treat more people
    b. Meeting other people with the same problem is frequently discouraging
    c. Groups are especially useful in treating problems involving social interaction
    d. Peer support may be more powerful than therapist support in increasing self-esteem

12. Encounter groups represent a group therapy technique developed by which type of therapy?
    a. Behavior
    b. Cognitive
    c. Humanistic-Existential
    d. Psychodynamic

13. Structural family therapy assumes that individuals develop abnormal behavior because
    a. their parents or siblings are abnormal
    b. of difficulties adjusting to family roles
    c. families encourage role experimentation
    d. the family unit is easily changed

14. A humanistic-existential therapist would accept which of the following as an appropriate outcome measure?
    a. reports of work supervisors
    b. direct observation of problem behavior
    c. changes in EEG and GSR measures
    d. client's report of how they feel

15. Which of the following is not of a problem of using meta-analysis to evaluate therapy?
    a. Poorly designed studies count as heavily as well designed studies
    b. Meta-analysis over looks differences in effectiveness between different therapies
    c. Many studies included in meta-analyses do not use real clients for subjects
    d. Scientific journals have a bias for articles showing psychotherapy has no effect

16. Your textbook suggests that, in general, research evidence suggests that psychotherapy
    a. is effective
    b. is effective for a limited number of individuals
    c. is not effective
    d. may be effective but we cannot tell from present evidence

17. Phenothiazines like Thorazine are used to treat
    a. anxiety attacks
    b. depression
    c. psychosis (hallucinations and delusions)
    d. sleeping disorders

18. ECT remains a controversial treatment for depression because
    a. there is no clear evidence that it is more effective than antidepressant drugs
    b. one of ECT's side effects is permanent memory loss
    c. it is not clear how or why it works
    d. all of the above statements are true

19. The nerve which joins the _____ and the _____ is severed in a prefrontal lobotomy.
    a. prefrontal cortex; frontal cortex
    b. hypothalamus; thalamus
    c. thalamus; prefrontal cortex
    d. frontal cortex; caudal cortex

20. Persons committed to a state hospital are likely to stay there
    a. for their lifetime
    b. for a legal maximum of 6 months
    c. until they can reenter society
    d. as long as they want

21. Deinstitutionalization has not been successful because
    a. funds were not made available for community based mental health programs
    b. people resisted putting community mental health centers in their neighborhoods
    c. deinstitutionalized individuals were not provided housing they could afford
    d. all of the above are true

TERMS AND CONCEPTS

Lesson 1
countertransference (529)
dream analysis (529)
ego analysis (530)
free association (528)
insight (528)
latent content (529)
manifest content (529)
modern psychodynamic approaches (529)
object-relations therapy (530)
psychiatric social worker (527)
psychiatrist (527)
psychoanalysis (527)
psychotherapy (526)
resistance (528)
traditional psychanalysis (527)
transference (529)
transference neurosis (529)
transference relationship (529)

Lesson 2
congruence (532)
dialogue (532)
empathetic understanding (532)
Fritz Perls (532)
genuineness (532)
Gestalt therapy (532)
humanistic-existential therapies (530)
logotherapy (533)
person-centered/client-centered therapy (530)
Carl Rogers (530)
unconditional positive regard (531)
Victor Frankl (533)

Lesson 3
Aaron Beck (534)
Albert Ellis (533)
Beck's cognitive therapy (534)
cognitive therapies (533)
rational-emotive therapy (533)

Lesson 4
assertiveness training (538)
aversive conditioning (537)
behavior therapy (535)
biofeedback training (538)
cognitive-behavior therapy (539)
covert sensitization (537)
eclecticism (540)
gradual exposure (536)
modeling (536)
operant conditioning (537)
self-control techniques (538)
self-monitoring (538)
social skills training (538)
symptom-substitution (536)
systematic desensitization (536)
token-economy (537)

TYING THINGS TOGETHER

1. Looking at Table 15.1 (page 543) of your text, discuss which factors each of the five types of therapy would assume are important to the effectiveness of psychotherapy.

2. For each of the five types of psychotherapy discussed in your chapter identify the outcome measure most appropriate for that type of psychotherapy.

3. Know that you have been exposed to both the theory behind the psychotherapeutic technique (Chapter 2) and the details of the therapeutic technique (this chapter), choose the approach to psychotherapy which you believe is the best. Next choose the outcome measure from Table 15.2 which you believe is the most appropriate goal for psychotherapy. Discuss any agreement or disagreement in your answers in light off your answer to question two, above.

4. Discuss the question, if there is no compelling evidence that psychotherapy is effective, should society continue to train psychotherapists and support their practice?

ANSWERS

Lesson 1
1 i
2 d
3 f
4 k
5 r
6 p
7 q
8 m
9 j
10 l
11 h
12 g
13 c
14 a
15 b
16 s
17 e
18 o
19 n

Lesson 2
1 i
2 j
3 g
4 a
5 h
6 d
7 k
8 f
9 l
10 c
11 f
12 b

Lesson 3
1 a
2 b
3 e
4 c
5 d

Lesson 4
1 d
2 j
3 b
4 m
5 n
6 k
7 f
8 h
9 o
10 p
11 c
12 i
13 e
14 l
15 g
16 a

Lesson 5
1 b
2 d
3 e
4 a
5 c

Lesson 6
1 k
2 f
3 g
4 a
5 d
6 c
7 i
8 h
9 e
10 j
11 b

Lesson 7
1 d
2 f
3 h
4 i
5 l
6 g
7 e
8 b
9 c
10 k
11 j
12 a

True-False answers
1 F
2 T
3 F
4 F
5 T
6 F
7 T
8 T
9 F
10 F
11 F
12 F
13 T
14 F
15 F
16 T
17 T
18 F
19 T
20 T
21 T

Multiple-Choice answers
1 d
2 d
3 d
4 c
5 b
6 d
7 c
8 c
9 c
10 c
11 b
12 c
13 b
14 d
15 d
16 a
17 c
18 d
19 c
20 c
21 d

16 Contemporary and Legal Issues

OVERVIEW

The major issues of this chapter, "Contemporary and Legal Issues," are legal ones. The first six sections cover legal obligations and conflicts for persons in helping professions. The last section covers two challenges facing helping professionals.

The first two sections, "Psychiatric Commitment" and "Predicting Dangerousness," examine two tasks which confront helping professionals. The first section discusses the conditions under which people can be committed or forced to receive treatment in psychiatric hospitals. One of the conditions necessary to commit people to institutions is that they be dangerous to themselves or others. The second section examines how reliably or accurately helping professionals are able to predict how dangerous people are.

The rights of patients in psychiatric facilities are covered in the third section of your text (Lesson 2 of this study guide). You will discover that individuals in the United States have a right to either receive or refuse treatment.

Your text continues with an examination of insanity. Insanity is a legal, not a psychological, concept. To say that someone is insane is to say that they are not legally responsible for their acts. Your text presents a brief history of the key legal cases which have led to the current controversy over insanity. There are two questions here that are still unresolved. Should insanity be a defense? And, under what conditions should we call someone insane? Although not a psychological concept, the opinion of helping professionals is often sought in making judgments about the sanity of an individual.

Insanity is one of two legal principles under which persons may not be held responsible for their behavior under the law. Incompetence is the other. A person must be competent to stand trial. After insanity, your text examines the principle of competence.

The last legal issue your text examines is a helping professional's duty to warn third parties of potential danger from a client. This duty to warn has been established by two court cases, one from California and one from Vermont. Your text includes an extensive examination of the pros and cons of requiring therapists to warn others of the dangerousness of clients.

The discussion of the duty to warn ends the examination of legal issues. While reading this material, you may begin to feel like you've stumbled into law school. In fact, you will need to do what a law student would do. Know the name of the case, the facts of the case, and the outcome of the case. You will notice that in covering legal issues, your text presents relatively few new concepts. Instead, your text covers those concepts and legal cases in considerable detail. You will need know those details.

Your chapter ends with an examination of two contemporary issues which confront helping professionals. The first is what to do about the large number of individuals who, because they are not dangerous, are being released from psychiatric hospitals even though they can in no way be considered "cured" of their abnormal behavior. You may find it amazing and disturbing to find that relatively little is being done for these persons. The second issue is how to prevent abnormal behavior from developing. Prevention is the primary focus of the emerging area of Community Psychology. Your text will examine some of the methods used to provide primary, secondary, and tertiary prevention.

CHAPTER OUTLINE, LESSONS & LEARNING OBJECTIVES

Lesson 1. The commitment and the dangerousness of the mentally ill. (563-567)
PSYCHIATRIC COMMITMENT (563-564)
1. Describe the legal procedures for psychiatric commitment.
2. Describe the development of safeguards to prevent abuses of psychiatric commitment.
3. Describe Thomas Szasz's objections to psychiatric commitment.
PREDICTING DANGEROUSNESS (564-567)
4. Summarize the research on predicting dangerousness by psychiatrists, psychologists, and others.
5. Explain how and why professionals overpredict dangerousness.

Lesson 2. The rights to receive and refuse treatment. (567-571)
PATIENTS' RIGHTS (567-571)
6. Summarize legal developments concerning the right to treatment.
7. Summarize legal developments concerning the right to refuse treatment.

Lesson 3. Abnormal psychology and the court room. (571-576)
THE INSANITY DEFENSE (571-576)
8. Summarize the history of the insanity plea.
9. Describe the term of commitment problem for perpetrators who are found insane.
10. Describe the problems of the insanity plea for jurors.
11. Describe the guilty-but-mentally-ill verdict.
12. Summarize Szasz's criticism that the insanity plea is degrading to the defendant.
COMPETENCY TO STAND TRIAL (576)
13. Describe the competency to stand trial principle.

Lesson 4. The duty of helping professionals to warn others. (576-578)
THE DUTY TO WARN (576-578)
14. Summarize the *Tarasoff* case and helping professionals' duty to warn third parties of threats posed by clients.
15. Summarize and discuss the controversy and conflicts surrounding the duty to warn issue.

Lesson 5. Preventing abnormal behavior and homelessness. (578-587)
FACING THE CHALLENGES OF HOMELESSNESS AND PREVENTION (578-587)
16. Describe the relationship between homelessness and abnormal behaviors.

17. Describe the needs of the psychiatric homeless population and discuss the multifaceted effort needed to meet them.
18. Summarize the philosophy of prevention.
19. Describe the three methods of prevention: primary prevention, secondary prevention, tertiary prevention.

Mastering Lesson 1. The commitment and the dangerousness of the mentally ill. (563-567)

This first lesson examines the three conditions under which an individual may be hospitalized in a psychiatric institution. These three conditions are civil commitment, legal commitment, and voluntary hospitalization. Hospitalization through civil commitment requires that an individual be judged dangerous to themselves or others with a fixed period of time, usually 72 hours. Hospitalization through legal commitment requires that an individual commit an illegal act because of mental disease or defect. This summarizes the basic concepts covered by your text in the first lesson.

This lesson does not require you to learn a large number of concepts. This lesson requires you to learn a few concepts very well and understand a complex set of issues related to those concepts. In particular, you will need to know the difficulties encountered in predicting dangerousness and why helping professionals overpredict it.

Match the following terms and concepts with the correct definition or description or explanation.

1. _D_ 72 hours
2. _C_ civil commitment
3. _B_ legal commitment
4. _E_ overpredicting dangerousness
5. _A_ voluntary hospitalization

a. a person can leave a psychiatric institution when they want
b. because a crime was due to mental disorder or defect
c. because a person is a threat to themselves or others
d. emergency power to hospitalize an individual
e. labeling people as potentially violent when they are not

Mastering Lesson 2. The rights to receive and refuse treatment. (567-571)

Mastering this lesson will require that you act like a law student. You will need to know the names of the four key legal cases discussed in your text. You will need to know the particulars (another name for facts) of each case and the disposition (another name for result). These four cases combined provide a detailed description of the rights of patients to receive and refuse treatment. Table 16.1 on page 568 of your text provides a partial list of patient's rights.

Like Lesson 1, the facts for this lesson are few in number. Your task in mastering this lesson does not end with knowing these facts. In addition, you need to understand benefits and costs of establishing these rights for patients.

Match the following terms and concepts with the correct definition or description or explanation.

1.__ O'Connor v. Donaldson
2.__ Rogers v. Okin
3.__ Wyatt v. Stickney
4.__ Youngberg v. Romeo

a. minimum standard of care for psychiatric hospitals
b. no involuntary commitment for persons who are not dangerous
c. psychotropic medications cannot be forced upon involuntarily committed patients
d. treatment for the confined in reasonable safety

Mastering Lesson 3. Abnormal psychology and the court room. (571-576)

Insanity, and the related issue of competency, are emotionally charged issues. Many Americans feel that it is unfair for people to "get away with it" when they commit a crime because they are insane or incompetent. One of the first things you will discover in reading the material for Lesson 3 is that these people certainly "get away" with nothing. They will spend a considerably longer period of time locked up than sane or competent criminals convicted of similar offenses.

This lesson examines the legal history of the insanity defense. You will again need to play law student. You will need to know the name of four cases, the particulars of those cases, and the disposition of those cases. You will also need to know the arguments pro and con for the insanity defense as well as attempts to limit its scope and reduce its impact. That is, you will need to understand the role of the American Legal Institutes guidelines for the insanity plea and the "guilty but mentally ill" verdict which has been instituted in some states. Likewise, you will need to know how long insane criminals are kept incarcerated and the conditions under which they may be released.

This lesson ends with a consideration of the competency to stand trial issue. You will need to know how competency and insanity differ and the effect of *Jackson v. Indiana* on how long incompetent individuals are incarcerated.

Match the following terms and concepts with the correct definition or description or explanation.

1. __ ALI guidelines
2. __ competency to stand trial
3. __ Durham v. United States
4. __ GBMI verdict
5. __ indeterminate commitment
6. __ insanity defense
7. __ irresistible impulse
8. __ Jackson v. Indiana
9. __ Jones v. United States
10.__ M'Naghten rule

a. a person can be committed until their sanity is regained
b. a person cannot be confined longer than necessary to determine competency to stand trial
c. a person is capable of understanding criminal charges and proceedings
d. claim of being guilty but mentally ill
e. claim of being not guilty due to mental defect or disorder
f. indeterminate commitment is legal for those not guilty through insanity
g. insane because of mental disease or defect
h. insane because one cannot conform to the law
i. insane because one cannot tell right from wrong
j. insane because one cannot tell right from wrong or because of irresistible impulse

206

Mastering Lesson 4. The duty of helping professionals to warn others. (576-578)

Lesson 4, and your text, is primarily concerned with a single court case, *Tarasoff v. Regents of the University of California*. You need to understand the particulars and disposition of this case. You also need to understand the dilemma that the disposition of this case poses for helping professionals. The intent of the court's decision in the Tarasoff case was to reduce the likelihood that a disturbed person would hurt another. You also need to now why the court decision may have inadvertently increased that possibility. Finally, you will need to know how the Peck case has extended the Tarasoff decision.

Match the following terms and concepts with the correct definition or description or explanation.

1.__ Peck v. Counseling Services of Addison County
2.__ Tarasoff v. Regents of the University of California

a. requires therapists to reveal confidential information to protect third parties
b. requires therapists to reveal confidential information to protect property

Mastering Lesson 5. Preventing abnormal behavior and homelessness. (578-587)

Your chapter ends with two problems for which there are no easy answers. There are many homeless Americans, many of whom have been discharged from psychiatric hospitals, not because they have been "cured" but simply because they are not dangerous. Your chapter discusses this problem and the difficulty in solving it. There are no concepts to be memorized here only issues to be understood. You will also need to know the research your text discusses, in particular, the research summarized by Figure 16-1 on page 580.

The second problem is the problem of preventing abnormal behavior. We do not encounter many of life's potential problems, because society has developed preventative measures which prevent those problems from occurring. The challenge of preventing problems has been taken up by the fields of health psychology and community psychology. You will need to learn with what these fields are concerned as well as some examples of and definitions for primary, secondary, and tertiary prevention practices for abnormal behavior.

Match the following terms and concepts with the correct definition or description or explanation.

1. __ primary prevention
2. __ secondary prevention
3. __ tertiary prevention
4. __ Community psychology
5. __ Health psychology

a. early intervention to prevent abnormal behavior from becoming severe
b. reducing the impact of abnormal behavior by providing rehabilitation
c. uncovering and eliminating the causes of abnormal behavior
d. the field which places a major emphasis on preventing physical illness by changing lifestyles
e. the filed which focuses using social systems to prevent and remedy abnormal behavior

PRACTICE EXAM

<u>Exam 1. (true-false)</u>

Indicate whether each of the following statements is **True** or **False**. Question numbers correspond to learning objectives from which the questions were drawn.

1.__ A person can never be hospitalized without their permission.
2.__ A civil commitment must be reviewed by a judge within 72 hours.
3.__ Thomas Szasz has argued for the elimination of civil commitment.
4.__ Persons who show abnormal behaviors are more likely than "normal" people to commit violent acts.
5.__ Professionals tend to predict a lower potential for violence among people with abnormal behavior than actually occurs.
6.__ Mental hospital patients have the right to suitable opportunities to interact with members of the opposite sex.
7.__ Patients in mental hospitals have a limited legal right to refuse treatment.
8.__ The earliest use of the insanity defense was the Hinckley case.
9.__ According to the Supreme Court in Jones v. United States, "there simply is no necessary correlation between the severity of the offense and length of time necessary for recovery."
10.__ Juries have the responsibility of determining if a defendant is insane.
11.__ The "guilty but mentally ill" verdict has reduced the number of "not guilty by reason of insanity" verdicts.
12.__ Thomas Szasz argues that the "mentally ill" should be treated like ordinary criminals if they commit crimes.
13.__ A person who is incompetent to stand trial is legally insane.
14.__ Tatiana Tarasoff killed her boyfriend after telling her therapist.
15.__ The Tarasoff decision has increased the precision with which therapists can predict violence in their clients.
16.__ Many homeless persons are involuntarily discharged mental-hospital patients.
17.__ Federal and state governments provided adequate community based facilities for persons released from mental hospitals.
18.__ Mental health systems in the United States are designed primarily to prevent abnormal behaviors from occurring.
19.__ Health psychology is the field which provides tertiary prevention for schizophrenia.

<u>Exam 2 (multiple-choice)</u>

Select the single, best answer for each question. Questions numbers correspond to learning objectives from which the questions were drawn.

1. A psychologist tells a judge that a person should be hospitalized because they are a threat to themselves. If the judge agrees and hospitalizes the person, we have an example of what kind of commitment.
   a. civil commitment
   b. criminal commitment
   c. legal commitment
   d. voluntary hospitalization

2. In Addington v. Texas, the United States Supreme Court ruled that a person can be involuntarily hospitalized
   a. if there are "mentally ill" alone
   b. if they are a danger to themselves or others alone
   c. only if they are "mentally ill" <u>or</u> a danger to themselves or others
   d. only if the are "mentally ill" <u>and</u> a danger to themselves or others

3. Thomas Szasz has suggested which of the following?
   a. Mental illness reflects and underlying medical problem
   b. People should not be deprived of their freedom simply because they appear different
   c. While the mental patient **is** dangerous; society **may** be dangerous
   d. Mentally ill people who violate the law should go free because they are not responsible

4. In a recent study conducted in Alaska, schizophrenics were found responsible for _____ of all arrests for violent crimes.
   a. a little more than 50%
   b. a little less than 25%
   c. a little more than 10%
   d. a little less than 2%

5. Professionals overpredict violence in people with abnormal behavior because
   a. they readily agree on what behavior is violent and dangerous
   b. behavior in hospital settings provide a good indicator for the community
   c. hospitalized individuals frequently issue specific threats to others
   d. violent acts in hospitals and society are relatively rare

6. Donaldson v. O'Connor established that a mentally ill person cannot be involuntarily hospitalized if they are dangerous to no one. While hospitalized, Kenneth Donaldson, the plaintiff who was institutionalized by his father,
   a. was provided with occupational training
   b. angrily refused medical treatments
   c. was a behavior problem on his ward
   d. received no treatment whatsoever

7. The right to refuse treatment
   a. has been established by the United States Supreme court
   b. is legally recognized in about half of the United States
   c. has been legally recognized only in the state of Massachusetts
   d. has still <u>not</u> been legally recognized in the United States

8. The first insanity defense in history established that a person was not guilty because of
   a. irresistible impulse
   b. the inability to tell right from wrong
   c. mental disease or defect
   d. inability to understand the crime

9. Michael Jones was caught shoplifting. A crime with a maximum punishment of one year in prison. He was found not guilty by reason of insanity,
   a. but was released immediately
   b. but confined to a hospital for six months
   c. and confined to a hospital for one year
   d. and was still confined seven years later

10. The ALI (American Law Institute) guidelines to define insanity, makes the decision of juries ____ because it ____ the number of cases in which the insanity plea could be used.
   a. harder; increases
   b. harder; decreases
   c. easier; increases
   d. easier; decreases

11. In the GBMI (guilty but mentally ill) verdict, the defendant
   a. is imprisoned
   b. can receive treatment
   c. may stay in prison longer because of the mental illness
   d. all of the above

12. Thomas Szasz believes that the insanity defense is degrading to defendants because it assumes that people
   a. have free choice
   b. lack personal responsibility
   c. have personal determination
   d. are guilty until proven innocent

13. If a person is found incompetent to stand trial, what happens?
   a. They are found guilty but mentally ill and confined to a prison
   b. They are confined in mental institution until they become competent
   c. They are immediately confined to a mental institution for life
   d. They are found not guilty by reason of insanity

14. One of the implications of the Tarasoff case is that
   a. it ended the principle of therapist-client confidentiality
   b. it created the principle of therapist-client confidentiality
   c. it requires the therapists to breach therapist-client confidentiality
   d. it requires clients to ask therapists about confidentiality

15. Requiring therapists to warn third parties of threats by their clients may increase the risk of violence by their clients because
   a. clients may become more willing to confide in their therapists
   b. potentially violent people may become more likely to enter therapy
   c. therapists may refuse too warn others because they resent this requirement
   d. therapists may be less willing to probe clients about violent tendencies

210

16. In a study of homeless persons in Los Angeles ___ of the homeless had shown psychotic symptoms in the past two weeks.
    a. about 40%
    b. more than 80%
    c. about 10%
    d. less than 2%

17. Persons released from mental hospitals require
    a. affordable housing
    b. alcohol abuse counseling
    c. social services
    d. all of the above

18. Which of the following is not an example of prevention?
    a. stock piling grain in case of famine
    b. genetic counseling for newlyweds
    c. getting vaccinated against polio
    d. releasing psychiatric hospital patients

19. Which of the following is an example of secondary prevention?
    a. suicide hot lines
    b. halfway houses
    c. communication skills training for engaged couples
    d. improved prenatal and perinatal care

TERMS AND CONCEPTS

Lesson 1
72 hours (564)
civil commitment (563)
legal commitment (563)
overpredicting dangerousness (564)
voluntary hospitalization (563)

Lesson 2
O'Connor v. Donaldson (568)
Rogers v. Okin (570)
Wyatt v. Stickney (568)
Youngberg v. Romeo (569)

Lesson 3
ALI guidelines (574)
competency to stand trial (576)
Durham v. United States (573)
GBMI verdict (573)
indeterminate commitment (574)
insanity defense (571)
irresistible impulse (574)
Jackson v. Indiana (576)
Jones v. United States (574)
M'Naghten rule (573)

Lesson 4
Peck v. Counseling Services of Addison County (578)
Tarasoff v. Regents of the University of California (577)

Lesson 5
primary prevention (581)
secondary prevention (581)
tertiary prevention (581)
Community psychology (586)
Health psychology (582)

TYING THINGS TOGETHER

1. Professionals tend to overpredict dangerousness. Write a brief essay discussing the benefits and costs of overprediction. Discuss the benefits and costs of reducing the amount of overprediction.

2. Imagine that you are your state's Director of Mental Health. Outline a program of prevention for the psychiatric hospital patients that you are discharging from your state's hospitals.

3. In a brief essay, explain why you believe (or do not believe) that your state courts should allow an insanity defense. What conditions should be met for someone to be judged insane.

4. Imagine you are a state legislator. You are about to vote on a bill which requires therapists to warn third parties of dangerous clients. How would you vote? Why?

ANSWERS

Lesson 1	Lesson 2	Lesson 3	Lesson 4
1 d	1 b	1 j	1 b
2 c	2 c	2 c	2 a
3 b	3 a	3 g	
4 e	4 d	4 d	Lesson 5
5 a		5 a	1 c
		6 e	2 a
		7 h	3 b
		8 b	4 e
		9 f	5 d
		10 i	

True-False answers

1 F	11 T
2 T	12 T
3 T	13 F
4 F	14 F
5 F	15 F
6 T	16 T
7 T	17 F
8 F	18 F
9 T	19 F
10 T	

Multiple-Choice answers

1 a	11 d
2 d	12 b
3 b	13 b
4 d	14 c
5 d	15 d
6 d	16 a
7 b	17 d
8 b	18 d
9 d	19 a
10 a	